MW00535448

Seven Peppercorns

Traditional Thai Medical Theory for Bodyworkers

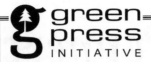

green
press
INITIATIVE

Findhorn Press is committed to preserving ancient forests and natural resources. We elected to print this title on 30% post consumer recycled paper, processed chlorine free. As a result, for this printing, we have saved:

6 Trees (40' tall and 6-8" diameter)
3 Million BTUs of Total Energy
514 Pounds of Greenhouse Gases
2,787 Gallons of Wastewater
186 Pounds of Solid Waste

Findhorn Press made this paper choice because our printer, Thomson-Shore, Inc., is a member of Green Press Initiative, a nonprofit program dedicated to supporting authors, publishers, and suppliers in their efforts to reduce their use of fiber obtained from endangered forests.

For more information, visit www.greenpressinitiative.org

Environmental impact estimates were made using the Environmental Defense Paper Calculator. For more information visit: www.papercalculator.org.

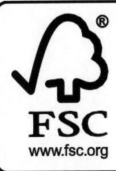

®

FSC
www.fsc.org

MIX
Paper from
responsible sources
FSC® C013483

Seven Peppercorns

Traditional Thai Medical Theory for Bodyworkers

Nephyr Anne Jacobsen

ILLUSTRATED BY
Rhonda Wheeler Baker

MAPS, COMPRESSES, & TREE
ILLUSTRATED BY
Serena Scaglione

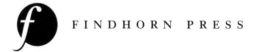

FINDHORN PRESS

©2015 Nephyr Anne Jacobsen,

The rights of Nephyr Anne Jacobsen to be identified as
the authors of this work have been asserted by her in accordance with
the Copyright, Designs and Patents Act 1998.

Published in 2015 by Findhorn Press, Scotland

ISBN: 978-1-84409-655-8

All rights reserved.

The contents of this book may not be reproduced in any form,
except for short extracts for quotation or review,
without the written permission of the publisher.

A CIP record for this title is available from the British Library.

Edited by Nicky Leach
Illustrations by Rhonda Wheeler Baker
Maps, Compresses, Tree by Serena Scaglione
Cover Design by Richard Crookes
Interior Design by Damian Keenan
Printed and bound in USA

Published by
Findhorn Press
117-121 High Street,
Forres IV36 1AB Scotland,
United Kingdom

t +44-(0)1309-690582
f +44(0)131-777-2711
e info@findhornpress.com
www.findhornpress.com

Contents

Part 2 - Roots of Thai Medicine

Dedicated to *AARON* and *DJANGO*,

for all the hours, the tromping around on the other side of the world,

the patience, and the love.

Dedicated to *TEVIJJO YOGI*,

for all the teaching.

And dedicated to *MOTHER EARTH* and *GANESHA*,

for a thing outside of words.

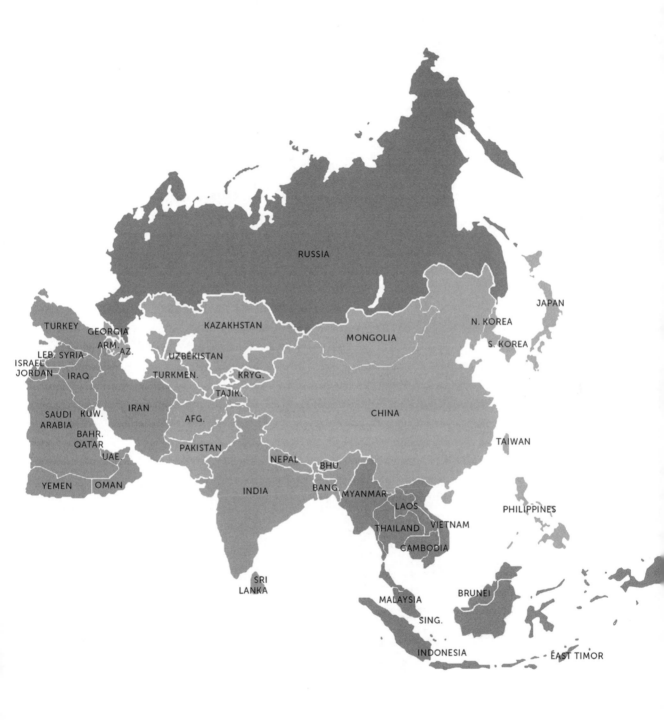

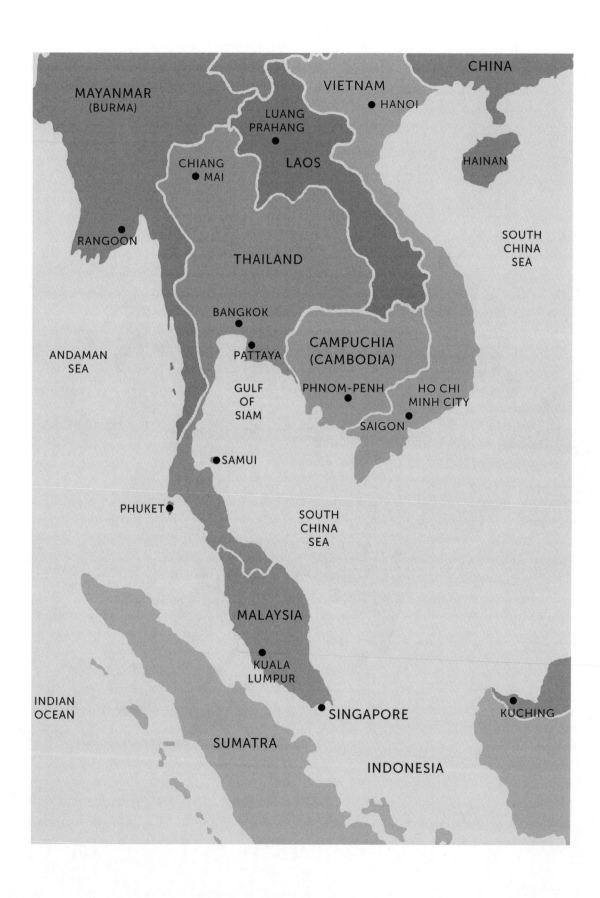

Preface

WHEN I WAS TWENTY-ONE, I took a two-week workshop at Harbin Hot Springs in California, in which we hiked naked in the woods, scalded ourselves in the thermal waters, and learned to give a very good Swedish massage. This led to following sky-diving events around the country doing massage at them (and occasionally plummeting out of little Cessna airplanes at high altitudes), which in turn led to falling off the road in Oregon, living in a crumbly shack on the beach, meeting my husband, going back to school, and becoming a licensed massage therapist.

Somewhere along the way, someone suggested that I go to Thailand and learn Thai massage. I knew nothing about Thai massage, but the suggestion found itself a cozy nook in my brain, where it made a nest and settled in, rousing itself from time to time to remind me that there was something I wanted to do.

Eventually, in 1998, Aaron (my soon-to-be husband) and I managed to go to Thailand, where I spent three months getting acquainted with the country and learning Thai massage, which turned out to be habit forming—both the getting acquainted with Thailand and the studying of Thai massage.

In the last sixteen years I have returned to Thailand time and again, including a two-year residency there, at first studying with many different teachers, then studying nearly exclusively with Pichest Boomthame[1] for a time, and finally focusing my studies with the man who came to be my primary instructor, Tevijjo Yogi. Tevijjo Yogi is a traditional medicine practitioner with vast knowledge of all aspects of the traditional medicine of Thailand. He began his studies of Thai medicine under the tutelage of a monk when he was in his early teens, and his lifelong studies and research, assisted by his ability to read archaic medical Thai, Lanna,[2] Pali, and Sanskrit, have made him an extraordinary expert on the subject.

It was Tevijjo Yogi who opened my eyes to what Thai bodywork really is, and the huge body of knowledge and practice that it is a part of. When I first met him I would ask him endless questions, to which he responded by letting me know just how many more questions I could be asking. I was requesting instruction on how to wade in a small pool, and he pointed out that there was the possibility of swimming in an ocean. And so for the last ten years I have been writing down, in a chaos of notes and computer files, everything that Tevijjo Yogi has taught me,

---

1   Pichest Boomthame is a well-known and rather amazing Thai bodywork instructor in Northern Thailand. His teaching is focused heavily on healing the healer and connecting with the spiritual through the Dharma. He is a physical therapies specialist as well as being to some degree a spirit doctor.

2   The ancient language of Northern Thailand, where older medical knowledge is well preserved.

whether we were in Thailand, Canada, the United States, or corresponding through e-mails, texts, and Skype from various points around the world.

This book is my attempt to herd those notes into a semblance of order so that I may share what I have been learning. I want to be clear that what I present here does not come from me. It comes from various medicine lineages in Thailand that have found their way from ancient times to now, to me, through Tevijjo Yogi.[3]

I don't always know when my notes are my own interpretation of Tevijjo Yogi's teachings, or were direct quotes, for when I took those notes I didn't know I would one day be turning them into a book. When I think of Thai medicine, my teacher's voice is so often in my head that the words that come out of my mouth may easily be stolen from his. And so, while the anecdotal stories are mine, as well as some bits of side research, I take no credit for the information presented here, although I do take full credit for any errors. Not everything in this book is from Tevijjo Yogi's teachings, but the vast majority of it is, and I owe the current level to which I am able to practice, teach, and write about Thai medicine to him.

It can be hard to express, in the writing of what is essentially a technical manual, the passion and the beauty, so I'll take a moment here to say it. Thai bodywork enfolds everything I have ever loved in any massage modality into one amazing system. Thai herbalism heals my family again and again, and gives me the tools to mend the hurts in my community. Thai medicine has led me repeatedly to the other side of the world, allowing me to witness pockets of an ancient and foreign culture as well as the modern tech happy world it is becoming.

My body is marked with the magical tattoos of a one-legged medicine man, and my life is marked in the invisible ink of encountering that which is different, until the strange becomes the mundane, a part of who you are, that which simply is.

Almost. For even when I was living in Thailand for two years there would be moments when I would look up while doing the dishes in our outside kitchen, where the water was whatever temperature the sky made it, and say, "I'm on the other side of the world . . . doing dishes!" and I would be consumed with the wonder of it. This is what Thai medicine has given me.

I watch as I teach classes at my little Thai medicine school, as Thai healing arts changes the lives of my students. I've watched Thai medicine lead people to change their careers, travel the world, learn a new language, open businesses, and embrace new spiritual practices. Because it is just that wonderful. So open these pages with me, like the doors of a little Cessna airplane. Feel the wind? You will learn as we free-fall through knowledge, that wind is movement, and that movement is what gives us life. Let's jump, shall we?

---

3   Throughout this book I will refer to him either as Tevijjo Yogi, or simply as "my teacher."

How to Use This Book

MEDICINE, INCLUDING TRADITIONAL THERAPIES such as bodywork and herbalism, cannot be fully learned from a book. Tradition emphasizes the need for a teacher in all walks of study; it holds that texts have never been intended to replace teachers, but rather to augment in person teachings and to remind us of what we have learned from our instructors.

Texts are meant to trigger the broader understanding that comes from a real-life teacher, and to expand on that teaching. Or, if you are reading an instructional book before taking a class, the book might prepare you for what you are about to learn, giving you a window into the subject such that when the real teaching begins, you know what you are walking into.

This is never more true than with a hands-on practice such as medicine. I will not attempt to teach you to be a practitioner in these pages, nor do I expect all of the techniques explained here to fully make sense without physical, three-dimensional guidance. How much you can utilize the information presented will likely depend on how much Thai bodywork or other healing arts training you have already have. Use care, and where things are unclear in print, seek out qualified teachers.

In this book I present Thai medicine as it has been taught to me: by practitioners for practitioners. I have done my best to leave my own cultural biases and beliefs out. Academics can argue about whether the Buddha really walked the earth, and scientists can debate the existence of spirits and ghosts, but this book is not written from or for the ivory tower. I present Thai medicine from the inside, not from the outsider looking at (and too often down upon) what those indigenous people "over there" are doing. This is from the dirt, from the floors of the healer's shack in the mountains, from the temples and the jungles. In Thai medicine there is no debate about the Buddha, for his teachings are a core of life. And there is no dispute about ghosts; they simply are. I present the information from this place of acceptance of how it is practiced and taught in Thailand.

In most Western countries, recipients of bodywork are referred to as "clients," for bodywork is viewed as a service along the lines of book keeping and facials. In the context of Thai healing arts, however, bodywork is medicine, and therefore those who receive it as such are referred to as "patients." This book will address those who come to you for healing work as patients, in the spirit of respecting that body therapies are a part of, and not separate from, other medical therapies.

This book is designed to be read straight through, as information builds in a linear progression. If you skip about and find that it leads to confusion, look for where a subject has been mentioned in other sections; the explanation you are seeking is probably there.

PART 1

Foundations of Thai Medicine

IN PART 1 OF THIS BOOK, we begin our journey into Thai healing with a foray into the past, establishing, to the best of our abilities, an understanding of where Thai medicine comes from, and its path to where it now stands. Knowing a bit of the history of our practice connects us with those who have gone before, allowing their knowledge to be passed down through the generations. It gives a fullness to our understanding, and an appreciation for the depth of time in which this wisdom exists.

From history we will move on to the daily practice of giving thanks and paying homage to the lineage and those who guide us; this, in turn, will lead us to the guidelines for Thai medicine practitioners. From here we will dive into the essence of the medicine: Thai anatomy and physiology. Here we get to explore the body and what animates it through the Thai medical lens of element theory. This is the foundation for everything that will follow, including the last section of Part I, in which we enter into the realm of disease and imbalance causation.

This walk through history, homage, anatomy, and imbalance lays the groundwork for understanding the material contained in Part II, in which we will see the therapeutic application of Thai healing arts through each of the five roots of the medicine. I hope that you enjoy your journey and gather many insights and a tool basket of practical skills along the way.

CHAPTER ONE

Getting Started

History of Traditional Thai Medicine

Early History

THE HISTORY OF THAI medicine begins and ends with the geographical region currently called Thailand. Tevijjo Yogi points out that:

> The indigenous practices of medicine and knowledge of the land and environment forms the basis of Thai medicine. This is true with any traditional medicine regardless of where it is from. The reason is, that which makes Thai medicine different from say Tibetan medicine or Malaysian medicine is the fact that the land is unique to Thailand/SE Asia (mainland), the climate is unique, the plants are unique and as a result the types of diseases and ailments one encounters are often unique.
>
> This is not to say that these medicines can only work here or that these diseases cannot be found any where else in the world. It only means that the disease process and the way in which medicines (properties of drugs) are used may differ from the same disease and/or medicine found in India, for example. We can see an illustration of this by looking at one type of orange grown in both Thailand and China. The exact same tree, when planted in China and Thailand yield completely different tasting fruits.
>
> The Chinese variety is sour and the Thai variety is sweet. It has to do with the difference in soil, air, climate, etc. If plants can experience such drastic differences, so can people... and they do.

It is important to keep this in mind as we move on to discussing the influx of various medical influences into the region. Hold on, through the convergence of many different people from many different places, to the knowledge that the heart of the medicine comes from the place it is practiced.

If we look at prehistory, we find that agriculture and metal work may have been developed in the area now known as Thailand, before anywhere else in the world.[4] I'm going to make an unscientific but obvious leap here and assume that where there is agriculture, people will have a highly developed relationship with plants. It is my belief that even before agriculture, in hunter-gatherer societies, an understanding of the medicinal abilities of certain plants is

---

4   Cummings, Joe. *Lonely Planet: Thailand*. 2005, pg. 32.

inherent. In *The Herbal Medicine-Maker's Handbook* (an utterly lovely book), herbalist James Green writes:

> *One can imagine how the first sparks of our vast herbal heritage were ignited. The inaugural attempts at the extraction of herbal properties were probably made soon after our deep ancestors discovered that certain plant materials were useful as food for nourishment, agents for altering consciousness, and medicines to alleviate physical and mental discomfort.*
>
> *Herbs collected for these purposes soon dried out, and it is logical to assume that our ancestral foreherbalists made attempts to restore the succulent qualities of these plants by steeping them in water. From this act, it was a simple step to discover that soaking plants in certain liquids dissolved the therapeutic powers of the plants and allowed their use in a more convenient, less cumbersome, and often more palatable form.*[5]

Just as where there are plants people will find ways to use their healing properties, where there are bodies, people will find ways to heal through touch; it is after all, the most natural thing in the world. If we go to a friend's house and find them sad, the first thing we do is lay our hands on them in a healing hug or comforting pat. It is medicine, an understanding of how cool reduces inflammation, when the injured hand is submerged in the stream. When was medicine developed in any region? When that hand first went into the cool stream and the inflammation went down. When the friend kneaded the hurt friend's shoulder and the ache reduced. When the leaf was chewed, and the stomach ache eased. Medicine is a natural discovery of humans, for it is a natural part of us.

This is why all over the world, we see the same techniques and theories in traditional medicines. For instance, cupping, a form of healing with suction, is found in the indigenous medicine of every continent on Earth and likely stems from the same impulse that leads a child to bring her injured arm to her mouth and apply oral suction.[6] The idea of the elements—Earth, Wind, Fire, and Water—being a part of our makeup and a part of healing is found from China to Greece to the Maya, and of course, Thailand.

To those who say that the stretches in Thai massage clearly show its origins in India due to their similarity to yoga, my teacher says, "Bodies bend the same all over the world." Seeing the same thing in two different places does not automatically mean they learned from one another (although, of course they may have). Healing is natural, and the plants around us, and our bodies themselves teach us what to do. In this light, to pick apart the origins of a culture's healing arts is in some ways unnecessary. Still, we are creatures who like to pull up the layers and see what comes from where.

The geographical region known today as Thailand, and previously known as Siam, is located in Southeast Asia, bordered by Malaysia to the south, Cambodia to the southeast, Lao to the

---

5   Green, James. *The Herbal Medicine-Maker's Handbook.* 2000, pg. 74.

6   Bentley, Bruce; from a 2006 interview conducted by Steven Clavey for *Health Traditions.*

east and northeast, and Myanmar (Burma) to the northeast and north. Other nearby countries include Vietnam, China, Sri Lanka, Tibet, and India. While Siam did not change its name to Thailand until 1939, for simplicity I will henceforth use the name Thailand regardless of the time period being discussed.

Most histories of Thailand tell that the people who came to be the primary inhabitants of Thailand are an ethnic group known as the T'ai or D'ai, who have been a distinct race for approximately 5,000 years.[7] Before inhabiting the region of Thailand, the T'ai people lived on the coast of Vietnam as well as central and southern China. (Most sources I have found list China as their place of origin, although it should be noted that they are a separate genetic group from the Chinese and have never been called Chinese.) Eventually the T'ai left, or were pushed out of these areas and migrated south into northern Thailand around 800 CE,[8] but we'll get to that in a moment. For now, the T'ai are still hanging out in southern China and northeastern Vietnam.

While the T'ai were up north and to the east, Thailand was occupied by the Mon (currently concentrated in Burma) and the Khmer (currently concentrated in Cambodia), and it is from these cultures that the first recorded evidence of medicine in Thailand comes. The use of herbal medicine is shown on stone plaques found in Khmer ruins, and while these mark the beginning of a record of medicine, the Mon and the Khmer were not the first to inhabit the region and therefore could not have been the first to formulate some sort of medical knowledge there. Evidence exists of people in Southeast Asia from between one and two million years ago (evidence of humans in Europe by contrast, does not appear until around half a million years ago),[9] so the history of indigenous peoples to the land is vast, even if documented records of them are scarce.

As a massage therapist, I've been subjected repeatedly to "groundbreaking" studies about massage or touch that come out from time to time from the scientific community—studies that positively prove that touch is good for you, or that infants require touch to survive.

I always laugh when I see these things. I mean, people have always known this, always. Most mothers know their children need pets and hugs and kisses and tickles. Who cannot see that rubbing your tired, aching shoulders brings relief? And to bring it back to the history of medicine in the land now called Thailand, I say that as long as there have been people, there has been medicine. They have been eating the plants and noticing the effects, they have been stretching their bodies, they have been touching one another. This "but of course!" statement tells us the true beginning of Traditional Thai Medicine. It is the same beginning as all medicines all over the world. It is exactly as ancient as humans—and in Thailand, that is very ancient indeed. Of what we know from historical records, my teacher writes;

Most of the history before the current dynasty, the Chakri Dynasty, is scarce and
hard to come by... Anything before the Khmer and Mon period is virtually unknown,

---

7   Gogoi, 1968, Wiens, 1967, Tregear, 1965, Eberhard, 1952, Carthew, 1959 and Benedict, 1975. As cited in *Ratarasarn, Somchintana.* 1986, pg. 4 (It should be noted that this "fact" is disputed and may be being dis-proven with current day research).

8   Salguero, Pierce. *Traditional Thai MedicineTraditional Thai Medicine*, 2007; timeline, prepagination.

9   Diamond, Jared. *Guns, Germs, and Steel*, 1997, pgs. 36 & 37.

although there has been evidence, by way of artifacts, of the medicinal use of various indigenous plants by the local people as far back as 5,000–10,000 years ago. Still, much of the history is unrecorded...

As for dates and times, it's really anyone's guess. What is traceable only dates back 1,000 years but the fact that there were hospitals and medicinal gardens illustrates the fact that there was a completely functional system of medicine in use far before this date.

By the time the T'ais arrived, the indigenous peoples of the land had been replaced by, or absorbed into, the Mon and the Khmer cultures. The previously agreed-upon idea that the T'ai people displaced the Mon and the Khmer and came to be the majority ethnic group in Thailand is not universally accepted these days, and it is possible that the Thai people of today are mostly descendants of the Mon and Khmer. These two cultures, having been heavily influenced by India, contained within them a mixture of Hinduism, Mahayana Buddhism, Theravada Buddhism, and Vajrayana Buddhism—all interwoven with the indigenous traditions of animism and spirit worship that predated Indianization.

In their time in Thailand, the Khmer's medicinal practices were advanced to the point of building hospitals; 102 of them were constructed by the Khmer king Jayavarman in the 13th century. It is logical to assume that by the time a culture is building hospitals it would already have a long history of medicine, and it is likely that at this point the indigenous medicinal knowledge would have intermingled with the medicine of India, as it rode into Southeast Asia in the saddlebags of Buddhism and Hinduism.

It bears mentioning that the medical knowledge coming in from India predates Ayurvedic medicine as it is practiced today, so it was not Ayurveda that was being folded into the mix of healing practices in Thailand but rather the seeds of the plant that would one day, in India, grow into Ayurveda. `These seeds grafted themselves onto the seeds in Thailand that would one day grow into the plant that is Traditional Thai Medicine. So while Ayurvedic medicine and Traditional Thai Medicine share certain similarities, they are not the same, and in actuality, Thai medicine more closely resembles Tibetan medicine than it does Indian. Some point to certain Thai medical texts that utilize a few words commonly found in Ayurvedic medicine[10] as indicators that Thai medicine is Ayurvedic; however, it must be understood that they are generally words that predate Ayurvedic medicine, stemming from ancient Buddhist medicine and the Pali and Sanskrit languages, and they do not always hold the same meaning when used in Thailand.

Just as the medical knowledge from India that came to Southeast Asia was not Ayurvedic medicine, the traditional medicine of India we see today, so trade with China brought not Traditional Chinese Medicine, as we know it, but the seeds that predate it. Again, this knowledge mixed with indigenous knowledge, the practices of the Mon and the Khmer, knowledge from India, and of course, medical practices of the incoming T'ais. This medical soup is the zygote of Traditional Thai Medicine as we now know it.

---

10 *Vayu, pitta,* and *semha* are examples of words found in both Ayurvedic and Thai medicine (the transliteration of the Thai for these terms would be *wâata ,bpìt-dtà, Săym-hà*), but only in more recent Thai medical texts, and only in a very few of them.

The incoming T'ais, like the Mon and the Khmer, practiced animism before their migration into the land now known as Thailand. Upon arrival, they adopted Theravada Buddhism[11] (primarily from the Mon), which mixed with the older tradition of animism, traces of which are still prevalent in Thai spirituality and medicine. This mix of Theravada Buddhism and animism was also flavored with the influence of Hinduism from the Khmer. Since religion was so thoroughly woven into the fabric of life, the development of medical practices was heavily laced with aspects of the religious/spiritual practices of the day. As Theravada Buddhism emerged from this mix as the most prevalent religious practice in Thailand, Traditional Thai Medicine can be said to be Buddhist medicine; in fact, the very foundations of Thai medical theory come from Buddhist texts and teachings.

Lanna Kingdom

In Thailand today, the peoples of northern Thailand make up a separate and distinct culture from mainstream Thai civilization. They call themselves *Lanna*, meaning "a million rice fields," or *Kon Muang* (คนเมือง), meaning "town people" (distinguishing them from the mountain-dwelling people back when Lanna culture emerged). Lanna culture predates Thai culture. It has its own written and spoken language (called Lanna, or Northern Thai), cultural traditions, and medical practices, which emerged from the T'ai Yuen people, the T'ai minority group that makes up the majority of Northern Thai demographics.

The heyday of Lanna culture began with the establishment of Chiang Rai by King Mengrai in 1262 CE, but existed for approximately 1,000 years prior to this. The Lanna Kingdom was for a long time the seat of Theravada Buddhism, preserving the Tripitaka[12] and many ancient texts; in fact, the oldest Thai texts extant come from the Lanna Kingdom. In addition to preserving various texts and Buddha dharma, Lanna civilization contains the least adulterated medical knowledge from ancient times, as a result of the Lanna people maintaining a degree of separation from emergent modern Thai culture.

From Sukhothai to Bangkok

The first T'ai capital was Sukhothai, where "medicinal gardens were established by the King in order to provide medicine for all the people of the kingdom."[13] It was not the first Thai city, however; cities such as Chiang Rai, Chiang Mai, and Lampun predate Sukhothai.

The time when Sukhothai was the capital is considered a golden era in Thailand. It lasted from 1238 CE until 1376 CE, when, according to Thai history, Sukhothai was destroyed by the Burmese. From here the T'ais moved south to create their second capital, Ayutthaya. While Ayutthaya would also be destroyed (twice!), some medical texts from this time have survived.[14]

---

11 A long history of nastiness with their new neighbors, the Mon and the Khmer, goes on to this day. Yes, even in Buddhist countries the arrival of new people can lead to the displacement of those that were there before, and subsequent bitterness and bloodshed.

12 These are important Buddhist teachings. *Tripitaka* translates as "Three Baskets," and contains the Sutra Pitaka, the Vinaya Pitaka, and the Abhidharma Pitaka.

13 Tevijjo, e-mail correspondence, 2008.

14 Salguero, Pierce. *Traditional Thai Medicine.* 2007, pg. 7.

They are scarce, and their existence at all is no small feat. Chris Baker and Pasuk Phongpaichit, authors of *A History Of Thailand*, describe the second sacking of Ayutthaya as follows:

> The Burmese aim was not to force Ayutthaya into tributary status, but to obliterate it as a rival capital by destroying not only the physical resources of the city but also its human resources, ideological resources, and intellectual resources. Any of these which were movable were carted away to Ava, including nobles, skilled people, Buddha images, books, weapons, and (reportedly) 2,000 members of the royal family. Resources that were immovable were destroyed. The walls were flattened and the arsenals trashed. The palaces and wats (Thai temples) that distinguished the city as a royal and religious centre were reduced to heaps of ruins and ashes.[15]

The primary medical text that survives from the Ayuthhaya period is *King Narai's Medicine*. This text contains formulas from a wide variety of doctors, including Indian, Burmese, Chinese, and even a couple of Western doctors[16] (we can see here that already the traditional medicine is changing with modern ideas). This was a book of medical formulas that would become the precursor for textbooks used even in today's Traditional Medicine degree programs in Thailand.

In addition to this text, many traditional medical formulas were recorded during the Ayutthaya period, as well as during the early emergence of Bangkok as capital after Ayuthaya's fall in 1767. And of course, there are practitioners who carry the orally handed down knowledge that spans across and beyond history. More often than not, and dating back long before a written language existed, the way that medical knowledge was carried on was from father to son, mother to daughter. Because of this, even with a dearth of written records, we can find an ancient medical tradition alive today in Thailand.

With the founding of Bangkok as the capital of Thailand, a cultural renaissance began. During this time, upon the grounds of an older temple, Wat Phra Chetuphon was built. Wat Phra Chetuphon, commonly known as Wat Po, was created to be a storehouse of knowledge, where the collected wisdom of the sciences of Thailand were chiseled into stone.

Here, as well as at Wat Raj Oros, there are to this day many medical formulas, charts, and statues that give us clues to ancient Thai medicine. Most of the medical statues existing today at Wat Po show *reu-sěe* (Thai ascetics that are a mixture of medicine man, monk, and shaman) in positions of the Thai self-healing system known as *reu-sěe dàt dton*.[17] The one remaining massage statue shows *reu-sěe* performing what appears to be a Thai massage technique. The *reu-sěe* are credited with the discovery of many healing practices in addition to a variety of other natural sciences. The depictions at Wat Po of *reu-sěe* performing bodywork on themselves

15 Baker, Chris and Pasuk Phongpaichit, *A History of Thailand*. 2005. pg. 23.

16 Tevijjo, e-mail correspondence, 2009.

17 It should be noted that the *reu-sěe* statues that augment the grounds of Wat Po are frequently mislabeled as statues of Jīvaka Kumārabhacca, another figure in Thai medicine who is discussed in detail later on page 31.

and others is a strong support for the oral tradition that credits the *reu-sĕe* with the creation/ discovery of Thai body therapies in addition to *reu-sĕe dàt dton*.

Recent History

Western influence upon Thai medicine began in the 1500s, with the arrival of Portuguese, Dutch, then British traders. American missionaries arrived in the 1820s (Western influence surged again in the 1960s with the Vietnam War). In 1890, the first modern medical school was begun in Siriraj Hospital, a hospital in Bangkok built in 1888 that exists to this day. At first, Siriraj Hospital taught both traditional and Western medicine side by side, but in an effort to modernize, the traditional medical curriculum was discontinued in 1915. Traditional medicine suffered, especially in urban areas, until the 1970s, when interest in the older ways of healing began to once again rise. The Ministry of Public Health began to promote traditional medicine, and continues to work toward the advancement, research, and standardization of traditional medicine to this day.

This is a double-edged sword, in that while standardization serves to preserve traditional medicine, it also decides what is and is not kept, leaving much out. With the governing agencies standardizing the medicine, there is also a tendency to focus on influences from Western and Indian sources, and, in an effort to appear scientific and modern, to cut away enormous portions of the medicine that are based on animism, Buddha dharma, and understanding of aspects such as ghosts, karma, and magic.

Modern-Day Westerners and Thai Massage

Western tourism began to have an influence on Traditional Thai Medicine, beginning in the 1970s. With tourists traveling to Thailand, the marketing of traditional medicine, specifically Thai massage, has become big business, and the practice of it is rapidly changing to meet Western standards and expectations. Seeking validation from the outside world, the Indian influence in Traditional Thai Medicine is frequently focused on to the point of negating or omitting all of the other sources. On top of this, travelers seeking to learn Thai medicine generally only focus on the bodywork component.

Thai massage schools catering to Westerners have become thriving industries in Thailand. These schools primarily teach techniques, with very little if any focus on medical theory. There are a few reasons for this that bear explanation.

Traditionally, medicine was not something that one could simply pay a school to teach you. Medicine had to be learned from a master, who might only take on a few students in his or her lifetime. And being a student was a serious commitment, requiring many years of apprenticeship and a lifetime of care and dedication to the teacher. So while Thais are happy to teach classes in Thai massage, there is an underlying cultural tradition that does not so easily offer up the deeper theoretical side of the medicine to visitors coming for short stays. And of course, the theory of medicine takes years to learn; one cannot fully learn it from a two-week class, or even a six-month course of study, as some schools are now offering.

Add to this the language barrier, and it starts to become clear that if you are not Thai, learning the medical theory of Thailand is a difficult endeavor indeed. Even learning medicine in the country in which you are born requires learning a whole new language: the language of anatomy and physiology. Imagine trying to learn this in a foreign country, where you are not fluent in the foundational language, let alone the medical verbiage. And with Traditional Thai Medicine, we aren't just talking about medical Thai, but archaic Thai and a form of Pali that even most Thais today do not speak.

Even if you were to overcome the language barrier, the odds of finding a true teacher and having the necessary years to commit to the study are very low. For these reasons, one cannot readily find Western practitioners of Thai body therapies who have had the opportunity to study the medical theory in depth.

Despite these obstacles, Western practitioners wish to share what they know and are inclined to offer classes and to write books on Thai massage. Of course, when they do this they are faced with a problem: their Western audience might want to know more than techniques; they might to want to know the theory behind the techniques.

Since there is almost nothing written in non-Thai languages about Thai medical theory, what most instructors of Thai massage in the West have done, therefore, is to turn to similar medical systems that have been written about extensively in Roman-based languages: Ayurvedic and Chinese medicine. Open just about any book on Thai massage that is written in a non-Thai language and what you will find is Thai techniques with an overlay of Ayurvedic or Chinese theory, most often Ayurvedic. While done with the best of intentions, this leads to the notio that Thai massage is not truly Thai. This idea has been perpetuated and spread to the point where one is now finding it being promoted by the Thais themselves.

As a result, a strange loop has been made, from Westerners learning in Thailand, taking the information home, altering and embellishing it, then exporting it back to Thailand. It is now possible for Westerners to teach Thai techniques with Ayurvedic theory and honestly say they learned all of this in Thailand. Fortunately in recent times ancient texts have begun to be translated, and thanks to my teacher, there is a small group of people beginning to record and teach Thai theory to those who do not speak Thai. This movement is in its infancy, but is sure to grow and bring new depth to Thai bodywork.

History Wrap-Up

While the influence of India upon the formation of Traditional Thai Medicine does indeed play a strong role in our story, it is important to remember that there are many primary sources of Thai medicine: indigenous practices and wisdom from those who lived in the land during its prehistory, Tibetan knowledge, China (pre-TCM), India (pre-Ayurveda), and the T'ai people, plus the Mon and Khmer influences. Fortunately in recent times ancient texts have begun to be translated, and thanks to my teacher, there is a small group of people beginning to record and teach Thai medical to those who do not speak Thai. This movement is in its infancy, but is sure to grow and bring new depth to Thai bodywork.

At the top of this list should be the indigenous practices, because, as discussed earlier, medicine is formed by the land. Climate and geography determine both the plants that grow and the diseases that will be prevalent. These multiple sources of Thai medicine can be seen in almost all traditional Thai medical practices, but how much of any source is present depends on the practitioner. Some practitioners incorporate more animistic practices, some bring in more of a Buddhist slant, and some have more of a Brahministic approach. Different people's prefer-ences, traditions, and trainings account for where they weight things.

In addition to our list of these ancient sources, we must consider that medical practices are not static. India, China, and the West all continue to develop their own medical practices and share them with the world, and Thailand too continues to develop its practices. There are still practitioners who follow the old ways of discovering healing methods, and from these old ways develop new medical formulas, mantras, and bodywork techniques. While these formulas and techniques may be new, they are also ancient, based on ancient pathways to understanding that can still be considered "traditional."

People like the *reu-sĕe* communicate with nature and ancestors to rediscover old medicine that has been long lost. Recently, my teacher said to me:

> *There is a real lack of knowledgeable people, and even the knowledge of the ancient wisdom. While there are many celestial (not physical) teachers around to help us, few are calling on them or listening to their advice. So now there arises a sense in some of us to go back to our roots. Go back to the wilderness. Live in harmony with the wild. this is the natural progression that is a result of the progression of society. Sooner or later, everyone will be forced into that position. If we choose to take it now, that's fine. We need to restore knowledge and wisdom of the ancients by taking nature as our teacher once again.*
>
> *However, we should never forget what has been left to us by the ancient sages and our ancestors. There is no need to start all over again. There is no need to toss everything away. We must preserve what is good and useful, fill in what is only partial knowledge, and learn as much as we can. We shouldn't put too much stock in the teachings of humans as most of their knowledge is tainted with desires for fame, name, wealth etc. We need to start by looking within ourselves. It's up to us to refresh and restore the knowledge of the ancients with practice, study, compassion, understanding, and diligence.*

Overview of Traditional Thai Medicine

Traditional Thai Medicine (inclusive of Lanna medicine) is made up of five primary roots that form the foundation for many different healing arts specialties. These roots are Medicinal Sciences, Physical Therapies, Spirit Medicine, Divinatory Sciences and Buddhism.

5 ROOTS
1. Medicinal Sciences
2. Physical Therapies
3. Spirit Medicine
4. Divinatory Sciences
5. Buddhism

These form a holistic blending of intensive physical/orthopedic therapies, herbal remedies, dietary and lifestyle counseling, divination, animistic spiritual healing, and Buddhist spiritual and lifestyle practices. Because Thailand is 95-98 percent Buddhist,[18] Buddhism integrates into all aspects of Thai life and culture, including traditional medicine. While you do not have to be Buddhist to practice Thai healing arts, Buddhism is woven into the theory and application to such a degree that an understanding of Buddhism is integral to the practice. The deeper you go in studying Thai medicine, the more it comes into play for, ultimately, while not all Buddhist medicine is Thai medicine, Thai medicine is inherently Buddhist medicine.

Underlying all roots of Traditional Thai Medicine, in addition to Buddhism, is Thai Element theory. Element theory is found in traditional medical systems the world over, and it is the connecting factor in every aspect of Traditional Thai Medicine. The idea that everything is made of Earth, Water, Fire, and Wind, with various balances of these elements creating harmony and disharmony within our physical, emotional, and mental beings, is found in ancient Mayan, Greek, Tibetan, Chinese, Indian, and Southeast Asian medicine, to name only a handful of medical histories. In Traditional Thai Medicine, element theory plays a central role, regardless of specialty or regional differences among therapists.

Just about any visit to a traditional doctor in Thailand will begin with the doctor discerning your basic core elemental constitution, and more importantly, what imbalances in your elemental makeup are triggering the complaints that led you to seek medical help. From this foundational understanding, the doctor will then apply his or her particular skills, be they in herbalism, bodywork, counseling, divinatory remedial advising, spirit medicine practices such as incantations and amulets, or Buddhist instruction in techniques to heal the mind, to assist you in bringing about elemental balance. For this reason, even if your primary focus is bodywork, it is important to have a foundational understanding of all five roots of Traditional Thai Medicine.

While the five roots of Traditional Thai Medicine must all be studied to some degree, if one is to be a holistic practitioner, it is not expected that you will specialize in all five. Just as a Western doctor must spend years studying all aspects of biomedical medicine—doing rotations in everything from internal medicine to obstetrics, even as they focus their practice on, say, brain surgery—a Traditional Thai Medicine doctor will have knowledge in all five roots, even as they hone their skills in, say, internal medicine or bodywork.

---

18 This figure will likely change in the near future due to the increasing numbers of Thai Christians.

These days there is a common misconception that a Thai massage doctor[19] only utilizes massage, and only has knowledge of massage. The reality is that bodywork doctors have extensive functional knowledge of the underlying theory that unites all five roots. The practice of Thai massage that is taught without theory and without knowledge in all five sciences is a modern evolution that has sprung from the street massage/tourist industry. Those who practice massage without theory are like massage therapists who do only spa relaxation massage and have not studied anatomy, physiology, deep tissue, myo-fascial release, or any other more therapy-based massage sciences. Relaxation massage has relevant application, but there is a difference.

Traditional Thai Medicine Specialties

In Thailand, a massage doctor will specialize in massage but will be able to use knowledge in all five roots to augment the bodywork. For example, the use of herbs in balms, liniments, poultices, compresses, and plasters is an area where we commonly see knowledge of herbalism complimenting a specialization in bodywork. Massage doctors may also use teas to help clear the channels or soften the tissues, or they may use astrological charts to understand a tricky elemental composition. They frequently use mantras and incantations to assist in healing. And of course, Buddhism is inherent in the work, everywhere from the practitioner's personal practices to working with a patient's mental well-being as it connects to healing the body.

Most writings on Thai medicine point out a difference between Royal and Rural medicine, sometimes calling the distinctions "indigenous and traditional" or "Court and Folk." In this text I do not make this distinction. Traditional medicine practices in Thailand have many variances, yet in reality these differences depend more upon the practitioner than upon the demographics in which he or she is placed. Those who practice in the rural village and those who practice among the city elite have more connection than separation between them, and a greater exchange of knowledge than the academics would have us believe. This said, there are rules that apply to working directly with royalty in Thailand that do not apply to the general populace, so any doctor, regardless of if they come from a city college background or a village family medicinal lineage, will have to adhere to these modifications in practice if working on royalty.

Thai medicine can be roughly broken into four practitioner categories: Thai doctors, traditional doctors, village doctors, and Lanna doctors.

For the sake of simplicity, this book uses the term "Traditional Thai Medicine" throughout. However, it should be noted that this is being used as a general term; it is not a reference to the first category above, and is inclusive of Lanna medicine. Used here as an umbrella term, it includes practices and knowledge from all the regional and government codified systems of medicine practiced in Thailand today. The information presented here draws from all four categories of Thai medicine.

---

19 Because Thai massage is part of the traditional medical system, in Thailand traditional medicine practitioners who specialize in bodywork are called "massage doctors," and the people they help are called "patients." Depending on where you live, this terminology might go against local massage regulations.

Four Practitioner Categories	
Traditional Thai Medicine (TTM) แพทย์แผนไทย *pâet păen tai* literal translation: *"Thai medicine"*	This is the most recent evolution of Thai medicine, having been codified in the 20th century and continuing to be modified in modern times. This systemized form of Thai medicine is taught at government approved schools. It stems from Bangkok, being promoted by the Ministry of Public Health and is taught in traditional medicine degree programs.
Traditional Medicine of Thailand (TM of T) แพทย์แผโบราณ *pâet păen-boh-raan* literal translation: *"Traditional medicine*	This system is based on texts dating back to the 1800s, written primarily in Thai and Khmer script. The practice of this system varies according to region, practitioner, and which texts are referenced.
Local Indigenous Medicine แพทย์พื้นบ้าน *pâet péun bâan* literal translation: *"Local Medicine"*	This category is likely the most pervasive as it encompasses local practices found throughout the country. Doctors who fall into this category utilize regional variations of theory and techniques, primarily predating TTM and TM of T, that are based on local texts and teachings.
Lanna Medicine แพทย์พื้นบ้านของลานนา *pâet péun bâan khawng laan-naa* literal translation: *"Local Medicine of Lanna"*	Lanna medicine is a sub-category of Local/Indigenous medicine. Lanna medicine is based on texts and teaching in the Lanna language. While there is much cross over between Thai and Lanna medicine, Lanna medicine is a separate system with ideas and techniques not found in mainstream Thai culture. The term pâet péun bâan khawng laan-naa,while accurate, is not colloquially in use, and local doctors prefer the term mŏr meuang (หมอเมือง)

Figureheads of Traditional Thai Medicine

The first time I met the renowned Thai massage teacher Pichest Boomthame, it was Thailand hot, air full of incense, altar full of flowers, the floor a chaos of Pichest's constant mess of offerings, papers, books, and cigarettes. Birds flew in and out of the open room, the occasional rat ran along a side wall, and roosters and dogs competed to dispel the myth of a quiet countryside. Pichest is a true master of Thai bodywork, a bit of a spirit doctor, and the most psychic person I have ever encountered.

I went to him at a time when I was chronically sick, a bafflement to doctors. I thought I was just going for the experience of getting a Thai massage from someone rumored to have greatness (this was before he became well known to Thai massage students the world over). I got this, but before he massaged me he performed an exorcism on me, complete with chanting, spitting holy water on me, and thunking me on the head a lot.

When Pichest was done with the chanting and hitting and spitting, he asked me in his broken English,"Who helping you?" I didn't really understand the question. I answered that I didn't know, and he sighed and told me to close my eyes.

Then he asked me again,"Who helping you?"Again, I said that I didn't know.

He told me to look, with my eyes closed, to see who is helping me, and I just shook my head as I tried and tried to reach for some answer to his question, which he asked me again and again, his voice losing a bit more of its patience with each repetition.

Tears of frustration gathered on my cheeks as I repeatedly said that I just didn't know who was helping me; I hardly understood the question. Behind my closed eyes I quested for the answer, feeling a despairing failure.

Pichest was finally shouting at me as he repeated his question and in a moment of pure frustration, my eyes still closed, I shouted back "I don't know. All I see is a herd of elephants!" Pichest immediately started laughing and laughing and laughing. I opened my eyes. I knew who was helping me, and I laughed with Pichest.

Ganesh had first come into my life in a dream I had when I was twenty-one years old, and had never heard of the elephant-headed Hindu god. I should have known the answer to Pichest's question right away, but I tend to panic and go blank when I feel tested, and so I searched and searched for an answer that was so obvious as to be presenting itself literally in herds.

This idea that we are being helped, that we do not work alone, is an important component of Thai medicine, and to truly incorporate it into one's healing practice takes more than simply recognizing that you have the support of, say, Ganesh. There are specific figureheads in Thai medicine who must be acknowledged, and with whom a relationship must be actively developed, if one is to have a traditional and complete healing arts practice. (I will address making this work for those who subscribe to a different faith later on).

The primary figureheads are The Lord Buddha, Doctor Jīvaka Kumārabhacca, and the *reu-sĕe* of old. In addition to these, you may have any number of specific ancestors, deities, angels, and spirits to whom you pay homage and nurture a connection. Great importance is also placed on acknowledging your parents and current life teachers. We must know that healing knowledge does not come from us alone, that regardless of who invented what, there are ancestors to be thanked, energies to be absorbed, help to be received. In this we do not work alone, but rather with the support of generations upon generations of healers. Here we will discuss the three primary figureheads of Traditional Thai Medicine.

The Buddha

There will be broader discussion of Buddhism in Chapter Eight. For now, I will take a moment simply to introduce The Buddha as a figurehead of Thai medicine.

Buddhism teaches that there have been four Buddhas to walk the earth, and that there will be one more. When people talk about the Buddha, they are referring to the Buddha of our time, Siddhāttha Gotama Sakyamuni, who is said to have lived about 2,500 years ago. He was preceded by Kakusandha Buddha, Koṇāgamana Buddha, and Kassapa Buddha, and will someday be followed by Metteyya Buddha. [20]

This probably raises the question, what is a Buddha? A Buddha is an enlightened person. However, Buddhas differ from other enlightened people in that they become enlightened at a time when all knowledge of the truth and the path to enlightenment has been lost—in other

---

20 Metteyya is the Pali spelling. The more commonly used Maitreya is Sanskrit. Since Pali is the language used in Thailand, throughout this book, when faced with a choice between the two, I have chosen to use the Pali spelling.

words, when there are no teachings for them to study and they must find the truth alone, without guidance. They then bring their enlightened knowledge to the world, sharing the truth through their compassion for humanity. And so we see that the fifth Buddha, Metteyya, will not come until all of Sakyamuni Buddha's teachings have been lost and forgotten.[21]

Sakyamuni Buddha, born Siddhāttha Gotama,[22] came from a family of wealth and prestige. It was foretold that he would grow to be either a powerful king or a spiritual ascetic. His parents, wishing the life of power for him, decided to shelter him from all things that might lead him to the spiritual life. Since spirituality often grows out of a quest away from suffering, they carefully insured that he did not learn of the harder side of life. He was raised in the family compound amid nothing but luxury, and at the age of sixteen he married Yaśodharā, with whom he fathered a son, Rāhula.

The story goes that eventually Siddhāttha left the family compound, and upon leaving it, he saw four people who changed his life. The first was a sick man, the second was an old man, and the third was a corpse. Sighting these first three taught him the reality of life—that we all are susceptible to illness, that we all age, and that we all die; that we all, in a word, suffer. The fourth person he saw was a spiritual ascetic, a man who had renounced the material world and made his way in rags and near starvation seeking enlightenment.

Siddhāttha was inspired by this last man to do likewise, so he left his family and gave up the wealth and luxury he had known until then. He joined a band of ascetics, and for many years engaged in practices of self-deprivation, including, so the stories tell, surviving on one grain of rice per day, becoming emaciated and weak. Eventually he lost faith in this path and left the other seekers to find his own way. There are many tales of both his time with the ascetics and his time alone, but I will jump us now to the story of the day he listened to a ferryman tuning his lute.

One day Siddhāttha sat by the river, emaciated and ragged. He heard a ferryman tuning a lute. One of the strings on the lute was strung very tight, and made a painful sharp sound. One of the strings was strung too loose, and made barely any sound at all. And the third string was strung perfectly, not tight or loose, and made a beautiful melodious sound.

Siddhāttha reflected on his life of luxury and his life of deprivation, and he saw how they were like the loose and tight strings, both extremes, and neither the answer to his quest for an end to suffering. From this experience grew his understanding of the Middle Way, a path that does not exist in extremes. This story, like nearly all stories of the Buddha's life, has many variations, and in some it is told not as an experience that Siddhāttha had before he became Sakyamuni Buddha but rather as a parable teaching that he gave after gaining enlightenment. Either way, the story holds a key aspect of Buddhism and the gentle approach it embraces.

Eventually, Siddhāttha decided that he would sit in meditation until he became enlightened. He sat underneath a Bodhi tree, some say for a night, some say for forty days. In this time he

---

21 It is thought that we are about halfway through this process of losing the teachings of the Buddha. The teachings are becoming corrupted, diluted, and mutated, but still have approximately another 2,500 years before being so lost as to require the birth of Metteyya.

22 Gotama is the Pali spelling. Gautama is the more commonly known Sanskrit spelling.

saw all of his thousands of past lives, and he came to see the Truth. When he came out of meditation he understood why people suffer and the way out of suffering. He was at peace, but at first he did not believe he would be able to share what he knew with others.

Siddhāttha was eventually convinced by the deity Brahma that he must teach people what he knew, and so began the Dharma. The Dharma is the teachings of The Buddha Sakyamuni. Of all the Buddhas that have come so far, he is known as the Great Healer because his teachings are focused on understanding why we suffer and on finding our way out of suffering. His teachings were inclusive of the mental causes of illness, medicinal understandings, knowledge of the elements, and knowledge of the body. His place as the first figurehead in Thai medicine is not only due to his role as a spiritual teacher but also due to this focus on an end to suffering, which is ultimately why we study the healing arts.

Jīvaka Kumārabhacca

Dr. Jīvaka Kumārabhacca is the founder of Thai medicine/Thai massage. He lived 2500 years ago and was the physician to the Buddha. The end.

Well, that's how it was originally told to me, and pretty much sums up the extent to which most people are educated about Dr. Jīvaka Kumārabhacca, also known as Doctor Cheewoke, the Father Doctor, and Doctor Shivago.[23] Here is the story as I tell it to my students, based on the original telling in the Pali Vinaya. I like to engage the storytelling aspect, so curl up with a blanket, a cup of tea, and enjoy.

Once upon a time in the fourth century BCE, there was a small city in northern India called Rajagaha. One day the leaders of this town journeyed to a nearby larger city in which there was an official city courtesan (high-class prostitute) whose job it was to entertain visiting dignitaries. The leaders of the city of Rajagaha found this tradition of having a city courtesan most delightful, and decided that their city should likewise have an official courtesan, whereupon they set out to find one.

And find one they did, in the lovely lady Salavarti. Trained in the arts of dance and discussion, she became the courtesan of Rajagaha and exerted herself to make the high-class guests of the city feel most comfortable. However, eventually Salavarti found herself with child. Knowing that this would not be an asset to her line of work, when the baby was born she ordered a slave woman to dispose of it. The newborn was wrapped in scarce cloth and thrown on a rubbish heap.

Fortunately for the discarded babe, his cries of abandonment were soon heard by a passing prince, who commanded that the child be rescued and brought to the palace. And so the baby was raised by Prince Ahhaya and named Jīvaka Kumārabhacca, said by some to mean "alive and raised by a prince." Others say his name means that he specialized in pediatrics.

When he came of age, Jīvaka Kumārabhacca decided that he wanted to study medicine, so

---

23 No connection to the 1970s movie *Doctor Zhivago*.

he traveled to the city of Taxlia, a thriving hub of medical education, where he had heard there lived a famous physician named Atreya, a rishi who played an important role in the history of medicine in India. In Taxlia he became Atreya's apprentice and studied with him for seven years.

At the end of seven years Atreya gave him the task of going forth around the city and bringing back all that was not medicine. After a long hard search, believing that he had failed, he returned to his teacher and stated that he could find nothing that was not medicine. Hearing this, Jīvaka Kumārabhacca's teacher pronounced him a true physician, done with his studies, and sent him off into the world to practice his healing arts.

At this point in the story, recorded in the *Pali Vinaya*, there are several accounts of Jīvaka Kumārabhacca curing various people, from merchants to kings, but the story of most notice to our tale is the story of him being asked to help the Buddha Gotama (Sakyamuni), who was feeling ill. In this tale, he aids the Buddha with gentle purgations, dietary changes, and lotus flowers.

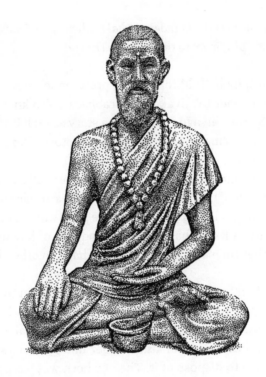

Other than just how cool it is to help someone as famous as *the* Buddha, this story is of importance because it began Jīvaka Kumārabhacca's relationship with Buddhism and the first sangha.[24] Following his care for the Buddha, Jīvaka Kumārabhacca became a Buddhist layperson, supporting the sangha through donations—most notably the donation of his medical services, which in time began a tradition of medicine in the monastery that has continued to this day.

---

24 A *sangha* is generally a community of Buddhist monks or nuns.

While this story is buried in an obscure Buddhist cannon regarding the rules of the sangha, and meant for monks to read, it somehow managed to be adopted into the healing traditions of many countries including Tibet, China, and Thailand, where in all three countries Dr. Jīvaka Kumārabhacca has become a legendary figure in the history of medicine. As the story migrated into the medical lore of different countries, parts of it remained the same, and parts of it changed to better fit its new homes. As stated by Pierce Salguero in *The Buddhist Medicine King*: "To translate is to rewrite."

In the Tibetan story,[25] Jīvaka Kumārabhacca is presented as the illegitimate son of King Bimbisara (Prince Abhya's father) and the wife of a merchant. In this version of the tale, the famous physician to whom Jīvaka Kumārabhacca apprenticed himself is named Atreya, the king of physicians, well known in Ayurvedic history, while in the original *Pali Vinaya* the physician is unnamed. Jīvaka Kumārabhacca learns from Atreya the art of trepanation (surgery in which the skull is opened), and upon leaving Atreya he comes across a gem that allows him to see inside his patient's body, illuminating the illness within.

In the Chinese version of the story, Jīvaka Kumārabhacca's tale changes more radically from its original. Here, he is no longer the son of a courtesan, nor is he the son of an adulterous union between the king and a merchant's wife; now he is instead the son of King Bimbisara and the divine virgin Amrapali.[26] Here, we begin to see clearly how the story adapts itself to the audience. To this point Salguero writes:

> *… certainly the combination of divine and royal parentage would have been more acceptable to Chinese audiences than either of the two extant versions.*[27]

Add to this the fact that in this tale Jīvaka Kumārabhacca is born with his fists full of acupuncture needles, and we can see our friend becoming a legendary figure of mythological proportions. In this telling, he acquires a piece of wood that, like the gem in the Tibetan version, allows him to see clearly the insides of his patients and thereby diagnose their disease.

In all three tellings of Jīvaka Kumārabhacca's life, numerous stories of specific healings are recounted, however only a handful of the healings are common to all three. Zysk sums up the similarities thus:

> *All versions contain an account of an operation involving the opening of the skull, or trepanation, to remove pain-causing animals. Similarly, the cure of one suffering from a knot in the bowels of twisted intestines by a type of laparotomy and the healing of King Pajjota (Pradyota) by the surreptitious application of the clarified butter are common to all versions.*[28]

---

25 Zysk, Kenneth. *Asceticism and Healing in Ancient India*

26 Ibid

27 Salguero, Pierce. *The Buddhist Medicine King*

28 Zysk, Kenneth. *Asceticism and Healing in Ancient India*

The famous healing of the Buddha, however, is different in all three versions. Again quoting Zysk:

> *Moreover, certain regional and doctrinal influences are highlighted in the Sanskrit-Tibetan account of Jīvaka Kumārabhacca's treatment of the Buddha. When all versions are compared, variations occur in the precise identification of Buddha's affliction. In the Pali account, it is a humoral disorder; in the Chinese, cold sweats; and in the Sanskrit-Tibetan, a disease characterized by chills and runny nose. When compared with the Pali, the Sanskrit-Tibetan version mentions the cold climate of the northern mountainous regions as the principal external cause of the Buddha's illness and relates a fourfold division with reference to the "peccant" humors (dosas), which are the internal causes. This association with cold climate is implied in the Chinese version. The predominance of four rather than three "peccant" humors is characteristic of Mahayana medical theory.[29]*

Certainly, just as Jesus is depicted with blond hair in North America, and Santa is brown-skinned in Africa, Jīvaka Kumārabhacca and the medicine he practices exemplify the characteristics and traits of the dominant culture telling the story.

As a student of Thai bodywork in Thailand, I see Jīvaka Kumārabhacca upheld as a sort of guiding spirit[30] of healing. There is a difference in Thai perception between ghosts, spirits, deities, demons, and teachers. Jīvaka Kumārabhacca would be a teacher, or *"khru."* As such, in terms of his wisdom, compassion, and power to heal, his spirit lives on through the various teachers and doctors who have practiced his methods or were influenced by him, but he is not a spirit in the sense of a being that hangs around to help us.

The guidance Thai healing arts practitioners receive from Jīvaka Kumārabhacca is in the form of the energy of healing that has been passed on down a long line of teachers. With Thai medicine practitioners, the day begins with a chant honoring Dr. Jīvaka Kumārabhacca, and a request that his healing knowledge be present with us in our work. He is held sacred in all of the healing arts, from village herbalists to biomedical doctors and dentists.

Because Westerners learning Thai massage are often taught only enough about Jīvaka Kumārabhacca to know that he is paid homage by Thai massage practitioners in Thailand, a few misconceptions have sprung up about him in the West, where it is easy to find websites and books that purport that he is the creator of Thai massage, that he was a monk or *reu-sĕe*, and that he traveled to Thailand where he taught the Thai people either Thai massage or all of traditional Thai medical theory.

To address the smallest of these misconceptions, it seems that Jīvaka Kumārabhacca was not a monk. It is likely that the assumptions that Dr. Jīvaka Kumārabhacca was a monk are based on his caring for the Buddha and his close association with the monastery. However, in those days monks were never doctors; he was more likely a white-robed lay Buddhist who sup-

---

29 Ibid

30 I use the term "spirit" loosely here. According to Tevijjo Yogi, Jīvaka Kumārabhacca is not, in fact, a spirit to the Thai way of thinking, but more like a *devata*, or heavenly being.

ported the monastic order through his donation of medical services—a donation that led to a long-standing tradition of medicine in the monasteries and very likely increased the numbers of people joining the monastic order. As a white-robed layperson, he would have taken higher precepts and practices than a regular layperson, without actually becoming a monk.

As for the idea that Dr. Jīvaka Kumārabhacca personally brought Thai massage and/or Thai medical theory to Thailand, Dr. Jīvaka Kumārabhacca never went to Thailand. His life was lived in India during the time of the Buddha, some 2,500 years ago, and it is only through Buddhist legends and texts, not through physical travel, that he arrived in Thailand. His influence as a figurehead of medicine, while very strong in Thailand, is not unique to Thailand and, as mentioned above, his story is told with local variations in Tibet and China, as well (he also did not travel to these countries as far as we know).

Lastly, to address the belief held by some that Dr. Jīvaka Kumārabhacca was the founder of Thai massage, it should be stated that while there are many detailed descriptions of medical services performed by Dr. Jīvaka Kumārabhacca recorded in the *Pali Vinaya*, there is not a single description of him doing any form of massage. Add to this the fact that there is currently no form of bodywork readily found in India that resembles Thai massage. On the other hand, there is a strong oral history in Thailand that sustains an understanding that Thai massage is indeed from Southeast Asia. It becomes ever more clear, therefore, that while the origins of Traditional Thai Medicine are debatable, it is likely that the massage component did not come directly from Dr. Jīvaka Kumārabhacca, or even from India.

For those who argue the clear Indian influences upon Thai massage, it is important to remember that influence is not the same as origin; it can come along and add to or shift things at any time. It is also notable that the honoring of Dr. Jīvaka Kumārabhacca is not unique to Thai massage practitioners. Healers of all sorts throughout Thailand, be they village herbalists, midwives, or even practitioners of Western allopathic medicine, such as surgeons, dermatologists, and dentists, honor Jīvaka Kumārabhacca. If we believe, based on the reverence with which he is held in the Thai massage world, that Dr. Jīvaka Kumārabhacca founded Thai massage, then we might also believe that he founded midwifery, allopathic medicine, herbalism, dentistry, and just about every healing modality found in Thailand today, as the doctor is equally honored in those professions.

So why pay homage to him at all? Well, just because he did not invent massage, this does not discount his important connection to the Thai healing arts. There are texts in the cannon of Thai medicine that are attributed to him, most notably those relating to children and childbirth. And in a Buddhist culture, just the fact that he worked directly with and healed the Buddha would be enough to warrant him thousands of years of homage.

Ultimately, Dr. Jīvaka Kumārabhacca was a great healer, and there is a level at which healing rises above the specifics of one medical modality or another. It is likely that he influenced Traditional Thai Medicine's theoretical system as a result of the knowledge that would have traveled to Thailand along with the spread of Buddhism and the relationship that grew up between medicine and monks and Jīvaka Kumārabhacca's healing work with the Buddha. While this is not the same as saying he created Thai medical theory, an influence upon it, even in a six-degrees-of-separation kind of way, is not insignificant.

In paying homage to Dr. Jīvaka Kumārabhacca, we are giving thanks for his great healing and asking that the energies of this esteemed healer be with us in our work, helping to guide us and protect us. In paying our respects to, and cultivating a relationship with, Dr. Jīvaka Kumārabhacca, we are honoring his role as a figurehead of medicine, not as the specific founder of the Thai massage lineage.

The Reu-sĕe
Reu-sĕe | ฤษี

Reu-sĕe are Thai Buddhist spiritual ascetics, a bit like a combination between a monk and a shaman, but with a different set of rules and purpose than monks. Monks generally live in a monastery, and it is their task to work toward personal enlightenment. In order to facilitate this, they separate themselves from the layman's world: they do not marry, have children, or jobs.

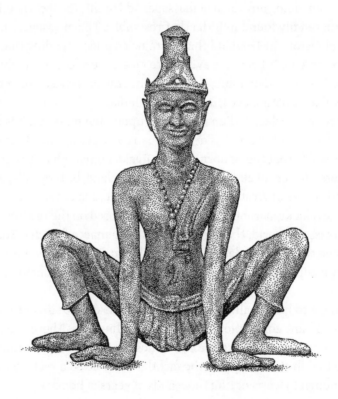

Reu-sĕe on the other hand, are more like Buddhist shamans, medicine men, or wizards, although some of this terminology is tricky, because while reu-sĕe are similar to the global concept of shamans/medicine men, there are shamans and medicine men in Thailand who are not reu-sĕe as they have different initiations, training, and precepts. These distinctions are further explained in chapter seven. Traditionally, reu-sĕe work to be in tune with the natural world, receiving wisdom from nature. As conduits of scientific knowledge such as the healing arts, *reu-sĕe* must work directly with laypeople. They do not have the same rules of separation that the monks have. While most *reu-sĕe* are hermits, technically they can marry and have children and work as teachers and medicine practitioners. The term "work" must be qualified, however, as they do not charge for their services, but rather depend on *dana* (donations voluntarily and joyfully given). The only work their vows allow is in the realm of teaching and healing; they cannot, say, be lawyers or bartenders.

Reu-sĕe study the natural sciences, including medicine, physical therapies, incantations, astrology, Buddhism, and even non-healing-related sciences, such as mathematics and music. They see themselves as the holders of the natural laws and sciences. My teacher, an initiated *reu-sĕe* himself, says;

> The term reu-sĕe in Thai is a blanket term for a variety of seers, ascetics, holy men, wizards, and other practitioners who choose to live and learn from nature and have the clarity of mind to receive her teachings. Of course, these types of people are all over the world in every tradition and in every culture, both men and women. they are the rishi of India, the yogis of Tibet, the Xian of China, the hermits of Europe, the Sufis of Islam, the shamans of the Americas and Africa... they are all of the same practice and the same fabric. Of course, all of these are unique and separate traditions, but they share many similar practices. The reu-sĕe of Thailand and Tibet are unique in that they follow the Buddhist tradition. While we interact with and respect nature just like the reu-sĕe in the world, we hold the Buddha and the dharma, which is the truth of nature, as the highest ideal and the highest truth. Some Thai reu-sĕe follow the example of the Sumedha reu-sĕe and take the Bodhisattva vow.

It is the ancient *reu-sĕe* who are credited with the transmission of much of traditional Thai medical knowledge, including Thai bodywork and other sciences. In truth, legend would attribute to the *reu-sĕe* of old, not to Dr. Jīvaka Kumārabhacca, the discovery of both self-massage techniques and assisted bodywork techniques, as found in Thai medicine, as well as the development of many ancient Thai medical formulas and protocols. Old medicine paintings often will show the image of the Buddha in the center, a *reu-sĕe* to his right, and Dr. Jīvaka Kumārabhacca to his left. This positioning of the *reu-sĕe* to the Buddha's right clearly indicates the *reu-sĕe's* high placement in medical history.

The question that arises from this is: If the *reu-sĕe* are more closely connected to the creation of Thai medicine, why is it Dr. Jīvaka Kumārabhacca that gets all the fanfare? I think there are two main considerations here. First, Dr. Jīvaka Kumārabhacca worked directly with the Buddha, and in a Buddhist culture this automatically brings him to the forefront of any figurehead hierarchy. And second, *reu-sĕe* are traditionally very hermit-like, preferring to live quiet lives in the forest, interacting with others primarily for the purpose of providing healing service or teachings. They keep to the shadows, so to speak. Even in Thailand, where there is still a living tradition and lineage of *reu-sĕe*, many Thais are unaware of their continued existence and believe the lineage to be dead.

I think that the general lack of awareness of *reu-sĕes* is accepted, and possibly even preferred by the *reu-sĕe,* as preserving the anonymity of the tradition; yet I also think that as a practitioner of Thai massage it is important to pay respects to this very important part of the lineage of Thai healing.

Today, interest in the *reu-sĕe* is on the rise in Thailand. While this has the nice effect of it now being much easier to find a statue of a *reu-sĕe* for my altar than it used to be, it also has produced people claiming to be *reu-sĕe* who do not have the proper training and initiation into the tradition. To truly be a *reu-sĕe* is a long hard path that requires an incredible commitment, a teacher, and certain fated events that are beyond the powers of an individual to create. Because of this there are only a handful of true *reu-sĕe* in existence in Thailand today.

Reu-sĕe are a bit different from Dr. Jīvaka Kumārabhacca and the Buddha as figureheads of Thai medicine, in that Jīvaka Kumārabhacca and the Buddha are individuals rather than a category of people, and also in that Jīvaka Kumārabhacca and the Buddha are both dead. It should be noted that in paying respects to the *reu-sĕe* in ceremony, and in developing a relationship with the *reu-sĕe* for your healing practice, it is the *reu-sĕe* of old, those involved in the origins of Thai medicine that you are incorporating into your practice. Of course, if you happen to have a modern-day *reu-sĕe* for a teacher, this person would also come into play in your homage, but it is different.

Other Deities

A Thai healer's spiritual practice will always recognize and incorporate the Buddha, Jīvaka Kumārabhacca, and the ancient *reu-sĕe*. In addition to this, an individual practitioner will often have any number of deities and spirits that they feel help them in their practice. In my personal practice, I pay homage to Ganesh and Mae Thoranee[31] as being deities whom I believe help me and to whom I wish to deepen my connection and give thanks. In Thailand, many Indian deities are brought into a healing arts practitioner's work, as well as the spirits of particularly relevant monks and ancestors. Thailand tends to be very open to any number of gods, goddesses, and celestial beings, always with Buddha at the center. Buddha, Jīvaka Kumārabhacca, and the *reu-sĕe* differ, in that they were humans who lived and died and are not considered deities, but the rules of spirituality in Thailand are painted in wide strokes to form a pantheistic picture.

---

31 Mae Thoranee is an Indian name for the Mother Earth goddess. Her image is found throughout Thailand.

The Wâi Khru Ceremony
ไหว้ครู

It is considered of utmost importance in the Thai tradition to have a teacher and to be initiated into the tradition, and to always honor and bring to mind our teachers and those who have come before us, when studying or using our knowledge practically. The reason for this is that there is a line, like a blood line within a family, that links us to the teachers of the past and allows us to invoke their knowledge and wisdom. It also gives us a form of protection being initiated into the tradition. By invoking the spirit of our teachers we are protected from negative influences and other unknown sources of harm such as ghosts, demons, black magic etc. It also gives us the power to heal those afflicted by these same things. For these, and other reasons, we always begin by performing the wâi khru.

— TEVIJJO YOGI

This was my first formal lesson with Tevijjo Yogi. It is the first lesson, because the *wâi khru* is considered the keystone to studying this art. The *wâi khru* is a ritual ceremony of gratitude offered to one's teachers: this includes one's parents, present-day teachers, teachers' teachers (and so forth up the lineage history), various possible deities, any deity or ancestor who is seen as the founder of your practice, and of course, (this being from Thailand) the Buddha.

In Thailand, one finds *wâi khru* ceremonies for nearly every aspect of life that includes direct instruction. *Wâi* means "respect," and is also the word for the posture of hands held together in prayer position that is used in showing deference and greeting throughout Thailand. The word *khru* comes from the Pali/Sanskrit word *guru* and means "teacher." So a *wâi khru* ceremony literally means to pay respect to one's teachers. More than just a time of giving thanks, it is a time to connect to one's teachers, and the teachers who went before them, as well as to the energies, wisdom, and protection that come from them.

Throughout Thailand, people in all walks of life perform daily, periodic, and yearly *wâi khru* ceremonies, each tailored to its individual purpose, depending on who is doing the ceremony and what walk of life they are treading. The way that the *wâi khru* ceremony is performed differs depending on the setting, but all pay homage to the Buddha; all give offerings of flowers, incense, and candles; and all ask that the performer of the ceremony tap into something older and wiser.

Schoolchildren gather once a year in the schoolyard for a *wâi khru* ceremony that honors (in addition to the Buddha and their parents) their current school teachers. They prostrate themselves before the teachers and give offerings of flowers, representing respect, patience, perseverance, discipline, and intelligence. Similarly, *muay Thai* (มวยไทย) kickboxers honor their teachers in an elaborate dance that leads the fighter to contemplate and thank his teachers, including the ancestral teacher seen as the founder of *muay* Thai.

Ceremonies such as this are endemic throughout the land. Musicians thank the founding teacher of music with sacred melodies; soldiers do a *wâi khru* ceremony similar to the *muay*

Thai fighters; and doctors, be they allopathic or traditional, practice *wâi khru* ceremonies like the ones encountered by students of Thai massage. It is this last one that I will elaborate on here.

Most non-Thai Thai massage practitioners have been taught at some point to do the *wâi khru,* whether they know it by name or not. A *wâi khru* practice is a bouquet of gratitude, blessings, protection, and connection. According to the Thai people, without it you can learn all of the Thai medicine techniques there are but you will not have learned the true healing. You will have only empty techniques with nothing inside them—nothing to give the techniques spirit, magic, mojo if you will.

Looking through the Thai lens, it is the *wâi khru* that gives the practitioner depth, divine inspiration, ancestral guidance, and protection. It is the substance behind the mechanics, for it is through the daily practice of giving offerings and chanting that one connects to the lineage of healing arts and nourishes relationship with protective and helpful deities. Again quoting Tevijjo Yogi:

> *Ideally a Thai massage therapist should perform the wâi khru daily, even on days when you will not be doing any massages. It's not about doing it just for those days (when you massage). Quite frankly, that's not enough. We don't stop being a student, healer, teacher... so, in order to invoke the spirits and teachers adequately it needs to be done every day. If you can't some days, it's no problem, but try to make the effort.*

My initial introduction to the *wâi khru* came at the first place I ever studied Thai massage. It was a well-marketed (even back then) school in northern Thailand that had a printed curriculum, air conditioning, and a large staff (yes, these things were remarkable then). Each morning would begin with the students chanting along to a tape recording of the director's voice saying the *wâi khru.* Because it was a recording, there was never the slightest variation in how the words were said. Morning after morning, for weeks on end, we said the *wâi khru* chant exactly the same, and the sound and cadence of that teacher's voice were forever burned into my memory. We didn't know the meaning of the words, nor the purpose of the chant, and there was something hollow in the taped rendition. We were told we should do this, but given no reason. As is so often the case with non-Thais learning the *wâi khru,* we were left to decide for ourselves what the meaning might be. Over the years I have heard some amazingly creative explanations.

Without a depth of understanding of the *wâi khru,* I quickly dropped it from my practice and left it behind until, first, Pierce Salguero and Pichest and, later, Tevijjo Yogi, came along, all to explain the ceremony to me in ever-increasing detail and expanding understanding of importance. Over the years, all of the teachers I have studied with have done the *wâi khru* ceremony somewhat differently from one another. Each teaches slightly, or dramatically, different words to the chant and a different way of approaching the ceremony. Some have required offerings; some have not. Some have had very short simple ceremonies; some longer and more elaborate.

Each *wâi khru* chant I have been taught has included an homage to the Buddha, an homage to Jīvaka Kumārabhacca, and generally an homage to the *reu-sĕe.* Most have included Buddhist refuges and precepts, and all have included incantations of healing. Each *wâi khru* has been chanted primarily in the Pali language, as Pali is to Thailand as Latin is to the Catholic church: it is not in common usage, but it is utilized in ceremonial chanting.

The *wâi khru* that I personally use—and the *wâi khru* that I teach my students—has changed many times over the years. It has been a particularly tricky bit of guidance from Tevijjo Yogi that every time I became comfortable with a new *wâi khru,* he would change a simple chant to a more complex one, add new homages, or confront me with new challenges in correct pronunciation. Over time, my *wâi khru* has gone from being the length of a few paragraphs to nine pages, when typed up, and back down to a few pages, as the time constraints of my life have led me to find a version that I can realistically incorporate into my daily habits. Following is a breakdown and explanation of a medium-length *wâi khru* healing arts ceremony. In Appendix B you will find this *wâi khru* without the explanation, for easier use.

Chanting should be done with the sound coming from as low in your belly as possible, in a deep strong voice. In Thailand, all words are considered to be sacred, and these words are especially sacred, so think about bringing these special words from deep inside you up through your body and out into the world.

When you first begin chanting, it is best to practice using a monotone cadence in order to learn proper pronunciation and rhythm. Once you are confident in your pronunciation you can play with more singsong chanting. Pay attention to commas, as they mark the natural pause in the chant. Many Buddhist concepts presented here are further elaborated in chapter seven and further instructions regarding Thai ceremony, offerings, and altar setup can be found just below.

Healer's Wai Khru	
Begin by lighting candles, incense, and placing fresh water and any other offerings you wish on the altar. Bow three or five times.	*Three bows represents bowing to The Buddha, the dharma and the sangha. Five bows adds bowing to your parents and teachers.*
Presenting the Offerings to the Triple Gem, Teachers, and Deities	*The triple gem is The Buddha, the dharma , and the sangha*
IMINĀ SAKĀRENA BUDDHAṀ ABHIPŪJAYĀMI, IMINĀ SAKĀRENA DHAMMAṀ ABHIPŪJAYĀMI, IMINĀ SAKĀRENA SAṄGHAṀ ABHIPŪJAYĀMI, (If chanting in a group, ABHIPŪJAYĀMI, is changed to ABHIPŪJAYĀMA)	*This chant dedicates your offerings to The Buddha, Dharma, Sangha, teachers and devas.*
Homage to the Buddha	*Bow once after chanting*
ARAHAṀ SAMMĀ SAṀBUDDHO BHAGAVĀ, BUDDHAṀ BHAGAVANTAṀ ABHIVĀDEMI	*The first three homages here (Buddha, Dharma & Sangha), together form the Homage to the Triple Gem chant*
Homage to the Dharma	*Bow once after chanting*
SVĀKKHĀTO BHAGAVATĀ DHAMMO, DHAMMAṀ NAMASSĀMI	*The Sangha represents those who have carried on The Buddha's teachings, and also any Buddhist community you are connected to.*
Homage to the Sangha	*Bow once after chanting*
SUPAṬIPANNO BHAGAVATO SĀVAKASAṄGHO, SAṄGHAṀ NAMĀMI	*The Sangha represents those who have carried on The Buddha's teachings, and also any Buddhist community you are connected to.*
Homage to the Parents	*Bow once after chanting*
MAYHAṀ MĀTĀ PITŪNAṀ VA, PĀDE VANDĀMI SĀDARAṀ	*This honors your parents for giving you life, and being your first teachers. It is not about the quality of your parents as teachers, or your current relationship with them. Some interpret this as honoring all beings, since it is a Buddhist belief that through many lifetimes all beings have been all things to one another, so all beings are your parents.*
Homage to Your Teachers	*bow once after chanting*
PAÑÑĀVUṬṬHI KARETE TE, DINNOVĀDE NAMĀMIHAṀ	*This honors your current life teachers, including influential people, guardian angels, deities, and spirits.*
Homage to the Buddha	
NAMO TASSA BHAGAVATO ARAHATO SAMMĀ SAṀBUDDHASSA NAMO TASSA BHAGAVATO ARAHATO SAMMĀ SAṀBUDDHASSA NAMO TASSA BHAGAVATO ARAHATO SAMMĀ SAṀBUDDHASSA	*This homage to the Buddha, like the homage to the Triple Gem is found in every true Thai wâi kru*

Healer's Wai Khru	
Taking Refuges	
BUDDHAM SARAṆAM GACCHĀMI DHAMMAM SARAṆAM GACCHĀMI SAṄGHAM SARAṆAM GACCHĀMI Repeat above with DUTIYAMPI added at the beginning of each line. Repeat above with TATIYAMPI added at the beginning of each line	*This chant essentially states that one goes to the Buddha, the dharma, and the sangha, for refuge (comfort, solace). It then repeats with Dutiyampi and Tatiyampi saying for a second time I go to the Buddha (dharma and sangha) for refuge, and for a third time.*
Precepts	*Precepts are promises to undertake a striving toward certain behavior or actions.*
1. PĀNATIPĀTĀ VERAMAṆĪ SIKKHĀPADAM SAMĀDIYĀMI 2. ADINĀDĀNĀ VERAMAṆĪ SIKKHĀPADAM SAMĀDIYĀMI 3. KĀMESU MICCHĀCĀRĀ VERAMAṆĪ SIKKHĀPADAM SAMĀDIYĀMI 4. MUSĀVĀDĀ VERAMAṆĪ SIKKHĀPADAM SAMĀDIYĀMI 5. SURĀMERAYA MAJJA PAMĀDAṬṬHĀNĀ VERAMAṆĪ SIKKHĀPADAM SAMĀDIYĀMI	• *The precept not to harm or kill* • *The precept not to take what is not given (all forms of theft)* • *The precept to abstain from sexual misconduct.* • *Meaning adultery, as rape and molestation are covered by the first precept* • *The precept not to engage in false speech* • *The precept to abstain from intoxication*
Presenting Offerings and Taking Refuge in The Teachers	
YAMAHAM GURŪPĀJJHĀYĀCĀRIYAM SARAṆAM GATO, IMINĀ SAKKĀRENA GURŪPĀJJHĀYĀCĀRIYAM ABHIPŪJAYĀMI Repeat with the word DUTIYAMPI placed at the beginning of the verse. Repeat with the word TATIYAMPI placed at the beginning of the verse	*This is similar to the first presenting offering chant, just with your guides/helpers in mind as the recipients of the offerings. It also affirms taking refuge in your teachers*
Homage to the Jīvaka Kumārabhacca	*Chant 3 times*
OM NAMO JĪVAKO, KARUṆIKO SABBA SATTĀNAM OSADHA DIBBAMANTAM, PABHĀSO SURIYĀCANDAM KUMĀRABHACCO PAKĀSESI, VANDĀMI SIRASĀ AHAM, PAṆḌITO SUMEDHASSO AROGĀ SUMANĀ HOMI	*Honors Jīvaka, praising him as being compassionate to all beings, a bringer of divine medicine, and shining like the sun and the moon.*
Homage to the *Reu-sĕe*	*Chant 3 times*
OM NAMASSITVĀ ISĪ SIDDHI, LOKANĀTHAM ANUTTARAM, ISĪ CA BANDHANAM SATTHA, AHAM VANDĀMI, TAM ISĪ SIDDHI VESSA	*Honors the Reu-sĕe of old*

Healer's Wai Khru	
If adding homages to personal deities, this is where to insert them	
Verses for Inviting the Teachers	*This chant is generally for the morning only*
VANDITVĀ ĀCĀRIYAṀ GURU PĀDAṀ, ĀGACCHĀYA ĀGACCHĀHI, SABBA KAMMAṀ PASIDDHI ME, SABBA ANTARĀYAṀ VINĀSSANTU, SABBA SIDDHI BHAVANTU ME	*This mantra calls the teachers (any beings and deities helping you) to be with you and to imbue your actions with powers, to give blessings and to remove obstacles. It should be recited with gratitude*
Verses to receive blessings from the teachers	*Can be done in the morning and/or evening*
SIDDHI KICCAṀ SIDDHI KAMMAṀ SIDDHI KĀRIYA TATHĀGATO SIDDHI TEJO JAYO NICCAṀ SIDDHI LĀBHO NIRANTARAṀ SABBA KAMMAṀ PASIDDHI ME AHAṀ SIDDHI BHAVANTU ME	*This is much like the mantra to invite the teachers in that it receives blessings of abundance, power and purity, and should be recited with gratitude.*
Acknowledgement of Faults	
KĀYA KAMMAṀ VACĪ KAMMAṀ MANO KAMMAṀ SAÑCICCA DOSAṀ ASAÑCICCA DOSAṀ ATĪTA DOSAṀ ANĀGATA DOSAṀ PACCUPANNA DOSAṀ SABBA DOSAṀ KHAMATHA ME BHANTE	*This mantra apologizes for any intended or unintended actions that have caused harm. It translates as:* *"From body actions and speech actions From mind intended and unintended In the past, future, and right now, may I be excused"*
Meditation of *Mettā*	*The first of the Brahmaviharas*
SABBE SATTĀ AVERĀ HONTU ABHYĀPAJJHĀ HONTU ANĪGHĀ HONTU SUKHĪ ATTĀNAṀ PARIHARANTU	*This is a meditation on loving-kindness, or good will toward all beings. It asks that all beings be free of enmity, ill treatment, and troubles of the mind and body, and that they have happiness.*
Meditation of *Karunā*	*The second of the Brahmaviharas*
SABBE SATTĀ ALĀBHĀ PAMUCCANTU AYASĀ PAMUCCANTU NINDĀ PAMUCCANTU DUKKHĀ PAMUCCANTU	*This is a meditation on compassion toward all beings. It asks that all being be free from loss, obscurity, blame and suffering.*

Healer's Wai Khru	
Meditation of *Muditā*	*The third of the Brahmaviharas*
SABBE SATTĀ LADDHASAMPATTITO MĀ VIGACCHANTU LADDHAYASATO MĀ VIGACCHANTU LADDHAPASAṄSATO MĀ VIGACCHANTU LADDHASUKHĀ MĀ VIGACCHANTU	*This is a meditation on sympathetic joy; sharing in happiness of all other beings. It asks that all beings have wealth, dignity, praise and happiness.*
Meditation of *Upekkhā*	*The fourth of the Brahmaviharas*
SABBE SATTĀ KAMMASAKĀ KAMMA DĀYĀDĀ KAMMA YONĪ KAMMA BANDHU KAMMA PAṬISARAṆĀ YAṀ KAMMAṀ KARISSANTI KALYĀṆAṀ VĀ PĀPAKAṀ VĀ TASSA DĀYĀDĀ BHAVISSANTI	*This is a meditation on equanimity; balanced, clear understanding.*
Verses for Removal of Disease	
UTTAMAṀ VARAṀ HITAṀ DEVAMANUSSĀNAṀ BUDDHATEJENA SOTTHINĀ NASSANTU PADDAVĀ SABBE DUKKHĀ VŪPASAMENTU TE SAKKATVĀ DHAMMARATANAṀ OSADHAṀ UTTAMAṀ VARAṀ PARIḶĀHŪPASAMAṆAṀ DHAMMATEJENA SOTTHINĀ NASSANTU PADDAVĀ SABBE BHAYĀ VŪPASAMENTU TE SAKKATVĀ SAṄGHARATANAṀ OSADHAṀ UTTAMAṀ VARAṀ ĀHUNEYYAṀ PĀHUṆEYYAṀ SAṄGHATEJENA SOTTHINĀ NASSANTU PADDAVĀ SABBE ROGĀ VŪPASAMENTU TE	*These verses wish for all adversities to perish, and all diseases and suffering to come to an end.*
Verses of Dedication of Merit and Aspiration	*To be chanted in the evening*
IDAṀ ME DĀNAṀ ĀSAVAKKHAYĀVAHAṀ HOTU IDAṀ ME SĪLAṀ NIBBĀNASSA PACCAYO HOTU IDAṀ ME BHĀVANAṀ MAGGASSA CA PHALASSA CA PACCAYO HOTU IDAṀ ME PUÑÑAṀ ĀSAVAKKHAYĀVAHAṀ NIBBĀNAM HOTU IDAṀ ME PUÑÑA BHĀGAṀ SABBA SATTĀNAṀ DEMA	*Just as the forgiveness chant above recognizes that we are bound to err, this chant recognizes that we are bound to do good. The dedication of merit offers up to others who may benefit from it, any merit you have earned through deeds intended or unintended. You can pour Water from one vessel to another while chanting it, and then pour the Water on the Earth outside when finished with the ceremony.*
Finish by saying **SĀDHU NO BHANTE** *and bowing 3 or 5 times*	Sādhu no bhante *means "well said"*

Application of the Wâi Kru

The wâi khru is ideally done on a daily basis by any practitioner of Thai medicine. While a person can do the wâi khru practice at any time, the best times are one hour before sunrise or one hour before sunset, as these transition times of day carry a special quality to them that is conducive to this sort of practice. The hours just before sunrise and sunset are times that are dominated by the Wind element, and so it is a time when connection to deities, spirits, ancestors, and the subtler energies that assist us is easier to establish. If a *wâi khru* practice is done in the morning, it is best to do it after bathing and using the toilet, but before eating, and it is important to brush one's teeth to have a clean mouth as this is where our words come from.[32] The *wâi khru* is generally performed before an altar with an image of the Buddha as well as images of any other teachers and/or deities being honored, however if no altar is available it can be done facing east. Having an altar with images of the Buddha and teachers is helpful in focusing our minds, but it is not the heart of the practice; it is merely a tool.

The *wâi khru* is performed kneeling, feet pointed back behind the body (toes curled under the foot for men). In Thailand it is considered impolite, especially for women, to sit in tailor position (lotus position, "Indian" style). Hands are held in prayer position in one of three places. They can be held at the level of the heart, with the fingers pointed up, thereby receiving energy into the heart, or the level of the throat, receiving energy into the throat, or at the forehead, receiving energy into the head.

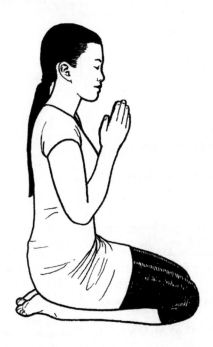

---

32 In Thailand, it is common for people to wear amulets with images of special monks, deities, or the Buddha. Because the amulets are sacred, you are supposed to remove them when you use the bathroom, especially if you are defecating. They should be placed on an altar, or someplace high up. I once asked my teacher what you do when you must use a public bathroom. He said, "Put the amulet in your mouth. Your mouth is sacred space." When I asked why this is, he said "Because your mouth is where words come from, and words are sacred".

Once positioned, the practitioner bows. The way that Thais bow in this setting is to begin with the hands in the prayer position close to the chest, elbows close in at the sides. The head is brought to the ground, with the hands above the head in prayer position, also touching the ground, so your arms and hands kind of make a triangle.

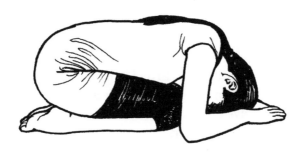

Because the idea of prostrating oneself before an altar with statues and other images on it is sometimes difficult for a Westerner to embrace, I would like to note here that the way it was explained to me is that one is not so much bowing to the statue of the Buddha, but rather to the qualities of the Buddha that one aspires to hold within oneself. The Buddha stated quite clearly in his teachings that he was not a god, and so it is not to a deity that one bows but to an image created to remind one of the teachings of a wise human. The same can be said of any images of Dr. Jīvaka Kumārabhacca, *reu-sĕe*, or other teachers that one may have upon one's altar. If you pay homage to any of the deities, such as Ganesh, Mother Earth, or Hanuman, as is often done in a *wâi khru* practice, this is a different matter, but I will assume that this notion of prostrating to a teacher or god or goddess is not an issue to you if you include deities in your practice.

In most traditions in Thailand it is standard to begin and end any ceremony with three bows—one for the Buddha, one for the dharma, and one for the sangha. In my training, we bow five times as we add a bow each for the parents and teachers. And also because the number five is significant in its relationship with the five elements, the five points of the human body, the five directions (north, east, south, west, and center), and the five Buddhas (four past, last one coming). Following offerings and bows, one chants the *wâi khru* chant of choice and finishes with three or five more prostrations.

Altar Arrangement and Offerings

Altars should face east, northeast, or north. So, if the altar faces east, then the practitioner would be facing west in order to face the altar. If you do not have an altar, simply face east yourself. Altars should be kept in a respectful place and be above waist height.[33] Images or statues of the Buddha are placed highest, farthest back, and centered on an altar. Images of Jīvaka Kumārabhacca and *reu-sĕe* go to the Buddha's right and left respectively, and are placed slightly forward. Other images, such as monks and personal deities, are placed farther forward, and can be slightly lower. Images of *nagas* and Mother Earth are traditionally placed much lower, closer to the floor (but not on the floor), as these are earth-dwelling beings. Offerings are generally placed on a separate level from the images of teachers and deities, although flowers can go anywhere and everywhere.

When in proximity to an altar it is important to be conscious of your behavior. Lower your head, do not point your feet at the altar, and avoid unharmonious speech, such as swearing or speaking ill of others. Traditional offerings given to the altar include: incense, candles, water, food, and flowers. Some also give tobacco, old money, alcohol, and fruit. Offerings should be made or purchased specifically for the altar.

Common items found on a Thai healer's altar include:
- Buddha image (usually a statue)
- Jīvaka Kumārabhacca image (usually a statue)
- Reu-sĕe image (usually a statue)
- Various deities, such as Ganesh, Hanuman, Mae Thoranee (Mother Earth)
- Images of important monks
- Images of the healer's personal teachers
- *Yantra* (sacred writings)
- Flowers - representing Space element or the order of monks
- Incense - representing Wind element
- Candles - representing Fire element, or two candles, represent wisdom and compassion
- Water - representing Water element or purity
- Food - representing Earth element, or simply the offering of food
- Tobacco, betel nuts, whiskey, tea, milk, old money - things are for the teachers of old who are thought of often as old men and women who enjoy these things. Alcohol on the altar is called *amirtra*, and is only offered in special circumstances. It receives the blessings from all of the chanting and prayer and is said to be good to drink when removed from the altar.

---

33 Anything below the waist is for baser practices, such as tattoos below the waist being for sexual attraction or overcoming others. These are considered lower arts. Working with higher energies requires elevating your altar and offerings.

Significance of Numbers in Incense Offerings	
1	Stick of incense is offered to ghosts
2	Sticks of incense are offered to parents
3	Sticks of incense can represent the Buddha, the Dharma, and the Sangha (3 jewels)
4	Sticks of incense are for the four elements or the 4 directions
5	Sticks of incense represents the five elements or the triple gem, plus parents and teachers
9	Sticks of incense represents the nine planets or the nine qualities of the Buddha
12	Sticks of incense represents the sun, all of the planets, constellations, a sense of everything
16	Sticks of incense are offered for all of the deities
33	Sticks of incense are for Indra's heavenly realm
108	Sticks of incense are for everything and should be offered on the Buddha days, outside

The question that often arises in relation to wâi khru altar offerings is why do we include alcohol, betel nuts, and tobacco when Buddhism clearly avoids intoxicants. The answer is that many of the gurus or deities on a Thai altar have distinct personalities that are honored. You give them things that they will enjoy. So, for example, a guru who is seen as an old man who lived a long time ago may be known to have enjoyed drinking and smoking. If the ceremony was purely in relation to the Buddha these substances would not be included, but because a *wâi khru* ceremony is not solely addressed to the Buddha there are allowances for things not purely Buddhist. The teacher-student relationship of the *wâi khru* is seen as separate from the Buddhist elements of the ceremony. Caring for those beings you wish to foster a relationship with is important. If Mother Earth is a part of your *wâi khru*, offer her incense and food, and pour water on the earth for her.

Most offerings can remain for several days, but water should be refreshed daily. Flowers can be left until they wilt, as this is a reminder of impermanence, although fresh flowers can be added at any time. Food and other offerings should be replaced when needed. New incense is burned daily, of course, as incense should never be extinguished but rather left to burn all the way down. Candles can be extinguished by waving a hand or snuffing, but not by blowing as blowing is seen as akin to spitting on the altar. One of the most important things about offerings is having a sense of giving them from your heart. It's not about how expensive or perfect they are, but rather about the sincerity with which they are given.

When offerings are finished, if possible put any edible substances that you do not intend to eat outside for wild animals, spirits, and ghosts. It is fine to offer unripe fruit. Leave it on the altar until ripe, then remove it for eating.[34] This avoids waste. Water from the altar is poured out on the earth, usually under a tree or plant. If you remove money from the altar it is good to

---

34 If you live in Thailand and have set up a spirit house, never eat the spirit house food.

donate this money to your teacher, or to some sort of charity. Altars are traditionally cleaned on the Thai New Year, which generally falls sometime in April.

Before removing items from the altar for the purpose of personal use, recite the following simple mantra three times:

SESAṀ MAṄGALAṀ YĀCĀMI
SESAṀ MAṄGALAṀ YĀCĀMI
SESAṀ MAṄGALAṀ YĀCĀMI

Visiting Thai Temples

If you visit Thailand you will find beautiful temples everywhere. In Thai temples, you interact more with the altar/temple than in other countries. In Thailand, you can go up to the altar and make offerings, chant silently, or sit in contemplation. Upon arriving at a Thai temple (a temple is called a *wát* วัด in Thailand), you will have the opportunity to get three incense sticks, candles, and flowers (and sometimes gold leaf). These items are usually provided for a small donation, or can be bought from vendors outside the temple. Take the offerings to the altar, light the candle and incense, and place the candle on the candle holder. Some people like to hold the incense and flowers while they say their prayers and do their prostrations, giving them to the altar afterwards, while others give them to the altar first; it can be done in either order. In the temple, you don't generally chant out loud, because they are communal places, but you can murmur or mouth your chant. If group chanting is going on you can usually join in, especially with morning and evening chanting.

Etiquette in a Thai temple requires that you remove your shoes before entering, and do not step on the threshold of the temple (it angers the resident spirits). Wear clothing that covers your shoulders and knees, preferably in light colors or white. Do not ever point your feet at the altar; you kneel facing the altar with feet facing back behind you, or sit with your legs folded to your side with feet facing back. Do not sit in lotus position in a Thai temple, as it is seen as indecently exposing your crotch to the altar. It is okay to take photographs in a Thai temple; just keep in mind that it is a functional place of spiritual practice, and be respectful of others who are there.

For Non-Buddhists

For those who practice Thai massage yet are faithful to a religion that does not have space within it for a Buddhist *wâi khru* practice, they can adjust their practice to more comfortably match their belief system. For example, prayers can be directed to Jesus, Allah, God, angels, Quan Yin, saints, Mother Earth, and so on. These prayers would be prayers of gratitude, and prayers for guidance and protection in your healing work. You should still be sure to give thanks for the lineage of training, your current-day teachers, and your parents. Atheists can spend a moment focused on gratitude for the handing down of knowledge, and tapping in to their own inner source of wisdom and self protection. These adjustments are fine for the average practitioner of Thai massage, but ultimately, the Buddhist spiritual component of Traditional Thai Medicine is integral to this healing system; to work on a deeper level with Thai medicine the Buddha's teachings would need to be embraced to some degree. Traditional Thai Medicine without Buddhism simply isn't Traditional Thai Medicine. Also, along these lines, there is said to be a strength to having a practice that utilizes chants or mantras that are used by others in the world. As my teacher says:

> This is the reason why certain incantations which are used all over the world, like Om Mani Padme Hum, have so much power; it's easier to use incantations which are used by many or used in groups in the beginning to effect a change. Sometimes it's hard to develop the concentration needed to use an incantation on our own.

Guidelines for Traditional Thai Medicine Practitioners

As is the case if you are a doctor, lawyer, or therapist, the practice of Traditional Thai Medicine comes with a set of guidelines, ethics, and study requirements. There are variations of the rules to be found, but the most basic are the ones put forth by the Ministry of Traditional Thai Medicine and the Buddhist precepts as they apply to a healing arts practice. In addition, it is expected that any healing arts practitioner maintain a study of the healing arts, as one is never considered to be done learning.

Traditional Rules Regarding Practicing Medicine

The Ministry of Traditional Medicine, a government agency in Thailand, has an official list of rules that massage therapists are expected to follow.

1. Do not drink alcohol

> ***Tevijjo Yogi says:*** *Of course, this includes any mind-altering substances. The idea here is that you must be clear-headed and able to make rational decisions. Some people say this only applies when you are working and others say you don't stop being a therapist and you never know when you may need to call upon your skills so you should always be in your right mind.*

You have to consider your skill set, as well. If what you know is how to give a relaxing massage, then you probably will not be called upon in an emergency, so occasional indulgence may not have the same consequences. On the other hand, if you know CPR, or other more advanced traditional or biomedical skills, then if you are in a situation where you would have been able to help someone if only you weren't intoxicated, there is a responsibility you will carry. Where I practice, in Oregon, all massage therapists are required to stay current in CPR and first aid, hence this would apply to all massage therapists, even if in their daily massage practice they do only relaxation massage and do not practice life-saving emergency medical arts. I am not presenting this as a personal judgment against those who sometimes imbibe, but to pass along the traditional view.

2. Do not engage in sexual misconduct

The actual Thai wording here is not to be a flirt, but since this word does not carry the same weight here, the meaning is really not to be flirtatious or use massage as a means of attracting someone romantically/sexually. And, of course, it also applies to not using massage for prostitution—giving sexual pleasure.

3. Do not deceive

This is about not leading people to believe that you have skills that you don't, or that you can heal them when you can't. Sometimes we don't know if we will be able to help someone at first, but if you can see that you are not helping, it is time to send them elsewhere—to allow them to keep giving you money for treatments is not honest. You must also be honest with yourself here and keep a clear head, so that you don't believe you are helping when you are not.

4. Perform massage only in appropriate places

Basically this rule applies to safety and intimacy. Safety is mostly about public places; if you are giving a massage in a public place, such as a fair or a trade show, there is a lot of noise and distraction. It is hard to tune in to what the patient's body is telling you, and the potential for injury is much higher. If you do massage at such events, it is important to keep the reason for this rule in mind and stick to simple massage techniques that are not dangerous. Overly intimate settings are also not appropriate for bodywork, as they can lead to misconceptions about intention. This applies to doing massage in hotel rooms, or in private houses, and especially in bedrooms.

5. Do not speak poorly of other practitioners or teachers

Of course, one reason for this is simply that speaking poorly of others is harmful and lacks compassion. But the reason that is less immediately clear is that if you go back far enough, you likely share a medicine lineage with the person you might be speaking ill of, so in a way would be hurting family.

6. Do not boast about your skills

This falls a bit into the same category as not deceiving, but even if you truly are a great physician, bragging about it is not beneficial.

7. Seek advice from your teachers

In this one we come to the idea that no matter how much you have studied, no matter how long you have practiced, and no matter if you yourself are a teacher, there is always more to learn. It is about having the humility to look to others for advice and wisdom, and to know that none of us have all the answers.

There are also a few more less official responsibilities of a traditional medicine practitioner, some apply to all, some it depends on your personal path. These are as follows:

- Uphold the five Buddhist precepts daily, and the eight precepts on full and new moons.[35] The precepts are further explained on page 223.
- Cultivate the four *Bhramaviharas*: the qualities of goodwill, compassion, sympathetic joy, and equanimity.
- Do your daily *wâi khru* ceremony, or otherwise honor your teachers and all who have brought you the knowledge you use. This is also found in our Western Hippocratic Oath as "To consider dear to me, as my parents, he who taught me this art."
- Give for free your healing arts services to renunciates, those who have chosen a spiritual path that forbids them from earning a financial living.
- Don't charge if you do not help. Also, if you have taken vows not to charge for your work, then of course, don't.
- Continue studying. There is no point at which you are no longer a student, even if you are also a teacher.

Studying and Practicing

Continuing to study and practice is what keeps our knowledge vibrant and meaningful. It is not enough to take a class on a subject, implement it into your practice, and be done with your education. To this end, if you have taken a Thai massage class and made the practice of Thai massage central to your work, it is important to always continue learning and bettering yourself in the art.

On the flip side, there are those who study but do not practice; often these are people who are inclined to teach. Teaching an art that you do not practice can only be responsibly done if it is in an academic, purely intellectual setting. For instance, if you do not practice Thai massage, you might teach it in the context of a class overviewing Thai medicine for intellectual purposes, but it would not make sense for you to teach it to people who plan to put it to practical use, actually doing bodywork on clients.

If you do not maintain a practice, you lose touch with the various potentials, effects, variations, dangers, and intricacies of the art. Those who have practiced for a long time and moved into a teaching position should still maintain some level of actual practice, even if it is just seeing a client here and there, or working on friends and family. And if you are learning new techniques and theories, it is imperative that you apply them yourself before instructing others.

Tradition teaches that the proper way of learning is to first listen to new information. Fully listen. Take some time to digest the new information, to understand it as best you can. Then ask questions if you have them. Listen to the answers, and again take time to digest what you have been taught. It is important to be able to be in student mode when learning, even if you yourself are a teacher. I have often seen people who take a class but cannot embrace simply being a student; instead, they take up class time showing others how much they know. To learn, we must

---

35 The eight precepts adds not eating after midday, not engaging in frivolous behavior, and not sleeping or sitting in high beds and chairs. It also changes the sexuality precept to celibacy for the time period that the eight precepts are being followed.

be able to remove our teacher hat, and enjoy the beauty of not knowing; we must embrace the Buddhist concept of beginner's mind. A long time ago, a wise man said to me, "Nephyr, relish your novice-hood; you only have it once." I think of these words every time I feel myself stumbling in new information, struggling to absorb, and feeling like a fawn whose legs don't yet work.

Traditionally, in Thailand, specific timelines were used to ensure that those new to a subject be sufficiently trained before they applied their skills to others. The traditional medicine study requirements are outlined as:

- **DOCTORS:** A minimum of ten years of study, apprenticeship, internship, and other practices. In Thailand, doctors were expected to also spend time as a monk before embracing the practice. Apprentice doctors might work as pharmacists, thereby gaining experience in the preparation and collection of herbal medicines.
- **MIDWIVES:** Midwifery was traditionally learned from a young age within a family. So a young woman whose mother was a midwife, might grow up learning the skills throughout her life. No set timeline was required because of the nature of the skills being passed down from parent to child.
- **PHARMACISTS:** Traditionally pharmacists would have three to five years of study and apprenticeship and would be expected to spend significant amounts of time living in nature learning directly from plants and animals.
- **MASSAGE THERAPISTS:** Traditionally, massage therapists would have at least five years of study and apprenticeship before they were considered ready to have their own professional practice. It must be understood that massage in this context is much more therapeutic treatment-based, an orthopedic physical therapy. Of course, a timeline like this would not make sense for a Swedish massage spa relaxation treatment; however, knowing this was the traditional amount of time required should give us pause and hopefully encourage massage therapists to dedicate more time to study.

These days, even in Thailand, these timelines are no longer adhered to. The modern-day official requirement for a pharmacist is one to two years, two more years are required to be a traditional doctor, one year of study is required for a midwife, and three months to one year for a massage therapist. This said, it is expected in Thailand that by the time you begin official schooling you will already have studied your practice a great deal through having personal teachers, often your parents. The entrance examination for the Ministry of Traditional Medicine degree program asks students to identify hundreds of herbs. This shows that the starting point of study is not what it appears. For massage therapists, many schools still require that you have at least five years of study and practice before you can teach.

Historically, books were not used as a primary way of learning a subject, but were instead used as reminders about a subject you are studying through direct student-teacher transmission and personal experimentation. Throughout Thai culture, there is a strong emphasis on honoring your teachers, making connection to your teachers, also making connection to your teachers' teachers, and so on through an ancestral progression. Having a real flesh-and-blood teacher allows for learning on a level that simply cannot be accomplished by reading books. Teachers can see where we are making unique errors or require adjustments to the techniques to accommodate our individual needs. They can assess our actual absorption of knowledge and adjust the method of instruction to better meet us where we are at in our learning process. Teachers also give us a kick in the pants when needed, not allowing us to be lazy or sloppy. In traditional medicine, a true teacher plays another less tangible role: they become energetic protectors, give us strength, and in some cases, continue to teach us even when they are not present. They also connect us to a line of teachers in a way that is difficult to accomplish alone.

This book is written with the knowledge that these days it is very difficult for people to find a qualified instructor in Thai physical therapies and theory if their goal is to go beyond basic, sequential, non-theoretical Thai massage. Even many of the well-known Thai massage teachers in Thailand, who are understood to offer the best instruction available to a Westerner, lack the ability to communicate the theory and more in-depth learning contained in these pages. This is generally due to language and time barriers, as well as knowledge protection and lack of a true student-teacher relationship. Still, as you read through this book, you are encouraged to try to find a teacher to work with, if possible, because ultimately, it is the best way to learn.

As you journey through this book, I recommend that you put into practice as much of the information as possible. If you are reading about the elements, try to go through your days thinking in terms of elements. Notice the heat of Fire from the sun, the stillness of Water in a puddle, the drying effects of Wind. If you are learning about tastes, go and find herbs in each taste category and taste them! It is important to have direct experience before applying your knowledge to your work on others. When learning bodywork techniques, seek out a qualified therapist who can use these skills on you, giving you a real understanding of their effects. Or seek out a class in these techniques where students will experiment on one another. It is through personal experience that we become the most skilled and empathic practitioners possible.

Gender in Practice

In traditional Thai healing arts practices, there are some modalities that are practiced by both genders and some that are customary for men only, or women only. For example, midwifery is a woman's art, whereas *yam khang*[36] is a men's art. The reason that midwifery is a women's practice is generally obvious, but Westerners do not always understand the reasoning behind certain healing arts practices being taboo for women to administer. In the case of spirit practices such as yam khan, it is generally believed that women are more vulnerable to possession, and so it is not a safe practice for them.

With spirit/magical medicine, there are two primary categories: practices that repel and practices that attract. Traditionally, women engage more in practices that attract while men do practices that repel. For instance, men will give protective tattoos and amulets, while women may give amulets that attract love or wealth. Women are more often found doing massage, cupping, and *tok sên*.

Traditionally women do not do healing arts when they are menstruating. The reason for this is that women are very raw and energetically open at this time and are therefore more likely to

---

36 A spiritual healing art used to drive out trouble-making spirits and energies.

take on the health issues, emotions, and energies of their patient. They are also more susceptible to spiritual possession at this time. Tevijjo Yogi says that practicing healing arts while you have your period is like going into a plague area with open wounds. This is not to look down on women; it's meant to protect them. The Thai word for "sacred" is *Saksit* ศักดิ์สิทธิ์, which comes from the Sanskrit words *Shakti Siddhi*, which means "women's power." Some practitioners will do bodywork on a menstruating woman and some will not, as some say that it is not good for women to receive bodywork at this time, and others acknowledge that bodywork can be beneficial.

Protection

Any healing arts practitioner must take steps to protect themselves from taking on illness, emotions, physical discomfort, and general maleficent "energy" from the people that they work on. Even those who intentionally choose the healing method of taking on other people's disease should do all they can to protect themselves from the ill effects. There are several traditional options for Thai therapists to work with:

- **PRECEPTS:** If you are a Buddhist (and, of course, in Thailand, nearly all practitioners are), the primary protection for all things is found in following the Buddhist precepts. Adhering to the precepts is said to bring peace to your life in many forms, including being protected.
- **WÂI-KRU:** One of the purposes of the *wâi khru* ceremony is to invite the energies/spirits/presence of your teachers and helpers to guide you and protect you. Doing a *wâi khru* chant every day, especially one that is inclusive of the precepts, is in itself an act of safeguarding your well-being.
- **AMULETS:** In Thailand, it is quite common to wear amulets as a form of protection. They often bear the image of the Buddha, a *reu-sěe*, an important monk, or a deity.
- **CLEANSING:** Cleansing as a form of protection is found in many healing arts traditions. Often, it is as simple as washing your hands in cold water after using them in a healing treatment session. In Thailand, they often infuse blessed herbs in a bowl of water and then dip their hands in the water, or splash it on arms and faces after doing healing work. The common herb for this purpose in Thailand is called *som poi*.
- **INCANTATIONS:** You can also cleanse a room in which healing arts are being practiced by saying the following mantra:

BUDDHAṀ PACCAKKHĀMI
DHAMMAṀ PACCAKKHĀMI
SAṄGHAṀ PACCAKKHĀMI

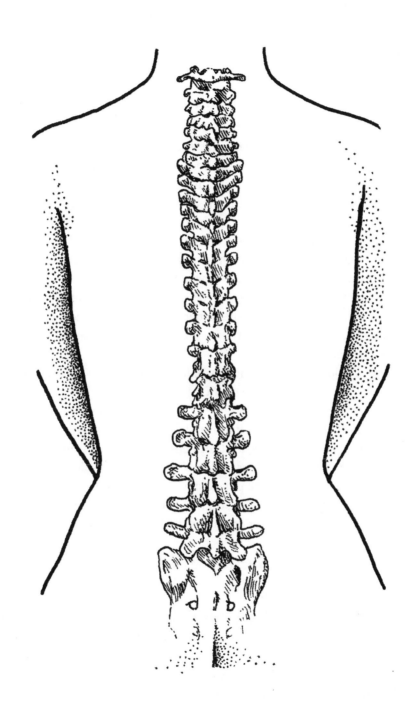

CHAPTER TWO

Thai Anatomy and Physiology

Introduction

FOR THE FIRST HANDFUL OF YEARS that I spent learning and practicing Thai bodywork, I thought that what made Thai massage Thai, what distinguished it from other bodywork modalities, was that it was performed on a mat on the floor, the client was clothed, and the techniques consisted of extensive passive stretching, thumbing of special lines on the body called *sên*, and compression. What I have come to understand is that none of those things are what make Thai bodywork Thai.

What makes the work Thai is the use of traditional Thai medical theory. If you are looking at the body as being made of Earth and Water, *sên* lines, Thai points, the 32 body parts, the 32 *kwăn*, the Wind gates, and the heart mind (all of which will be explained in this chapter), and if you are understanding that the body is animated by Fire and Wind, then your approach to the body will be Thai. If you are using Thai element theory, Thai *sên* line theory, Thai point theory, and Thai understanding of dis-ease causation to guide your choices and actions, then you are going to be doing Thai bodywork.

This may not always look like what most people associate with Thai massage. Using Thai anatomy, physiology, and traditional Thai medical theory, you may decide that someone with a Wind imbalance needs to have sesame oil rubbed all over their body. To an outsider watching, what you are doing may look an awful lot like Swedish massage, but ultimately what makes the modality Thai isn't outside appearances; it's the deeper knowledge of the theory, and the ability to look at your patient through the lens of Thai anatomy and physiology.

What do I mean by Thai anatomy and physiology? I mean how Thai medicine practitioners see that which makes up our physical being, that which animates us, and that which makes up the subtler realities of us, such as our thoughts and feelings. Let's take a close look.

Thai Element Theory

Overview of Thai Element Theory

Traditional Thai Medicine has five different roots: Medicinal Sciences, Physical Therapies, Spirit Medicine, Divinatory Sciences, and Buddhism (which can be seen as the mental health root). These roots are bound together by two common threads: Buddhist concepts and view, and Thai element theory. Element theory is the foundation of all Traditional Thai Medicine, regardless of regional variations, medicinal specialization, or stylistic preferences. To learn any aspect of Traditional Thai Medicine without learning element theory is to not truly learn that aspect. It is the unique focus of Thai medicine; it is what binds all aspects of Thai medicine together; and it is the basis upon which all traditional Thai medical diagnosis and treatments are founded.

In *The Principles and Concepts of Thai Classical Medicine* by Somchintana Ratarasarn, she states:

> The concept of the Four Body Elements emically explains every part, both physiological and non-physiological, of the human body. Hence it is a must for an orthodox Thai doctor to have knowledge in the four Body Elements before he can cure his patients by prescribing any medicine, mode and degree of treatment.
>
> The basic principle of every branch of Thai ethnomedicine, particularly internal medicine, is the knowledge of the Four Body Elements, their functions and their interrelations which affect the health/sickness of the individual. The Four Body Elements are regarded as "The foundation of the whole body and the foundation of life and durability.

Element theory holds that everything from the ground we walk on to the food we eat, from our bones to our thoughts, is made up of the elements Earth (*tâat Din* ธาตุดิน), Water (*tâat Nám* ธาตุน้ำ), Fire (*tâat Fai* ธาตุไฟ), Wind (*tâat Lom* ธาตุลม), and Space (*Aa-gàat tâat* อากาศธาตุ). It is the balance, or imbalance of these elements within us that is the root cause of all health and disease. Element theory is not unique to Thailand, being found in the traditional medicine of China, India, ancient Greece, Maya, and many other cultures; however, it is perhaps uniquely central in its importance in Traditional Thai Medicine, for the elements truly are the heart and soul of this healing system.

When we look at the world seeing elements, we see that the wind blowing through the trees bringing motion to the leaves is the same element that we inhale, the same elemental qualities that animate us. We see that the qualities of solidity and structure that make up the earth that we walk on, the earth that is a boulder or a flat of desert sand, that these are the same Earth element qualities that make up our bones and teeth. We see that the fluid nature of the water that flows in the rivers, the water that is the moisture in a juicy mango is the same fluid nature as the water of our tears and sweat.

When we can see this, we can begin to understand how medicine works. Through this lens, it makes sense that plants, being made of the same building blocks that we are made of, would have a *simpatico* relationship with our bodies and be able to bring about balance and healing; or, if used incorrectly, bring about imbalance and illness. Comprehending this, we can understand how a person depleted of Fire, weak and fatigued, can be nourished by absorbing the warming rays of the sun, and we can make the connection between an inflamed injury and the therapy of a wash cloth soaked in cooling water.

The primary elements that are used in Traditional Thai Medicine are Earth, Water, Fire, and Wind. A practitioner who focuses on these four elements would be using Four Element theory. A practitioner who also focuses on Space, is using Five Element theory. In addition to this, some people count Consciousness (*win-yaana tâat* วิญญาณธาตุ) as a sixth element, thereby using Six Element theory.[37] All practitioners of Traditional Thai Medicine recognize the existence of all

---

37 This is found more prevalently in Lanna medicine.

six elements, but many group Space and Consciousness together, and many only utilize Four Element theory in their work focusing on Earth, Water, Fire, and Wind.

While the elements are the component parts of everything, the building blocks of all matter, it is important to realize that they do not exist in all things in equal states. While there is water in even a rock (the rock would crumble to dust without it), the rock has far more excited Earth element than Water element. Likewise an orange has excited Water element in it, but clearly is not entirely Water. Our bodies also are made up of all of the elements, but different parts of our anatomy naturally have one element more excited than the others. Our bones, for example, are excited Earth element, while our synovial fluid is amplified Water. Our thoughts and motions are more Wind, while our metabolic processes, body heat, and motivation are more Fire. Wind and Fire are not tangible forces in the same way as Earth and Water, but rather are the elements that animate us, and they too exist in varying states.

Learning to see the elements in the world around us, as well as within those we live with and hope to bring healing to, is essential to any Thai medicine practice, including Thai bodywork. The following paragraphs and tables provide an overview of each of the five elements, as well as tools for connecting to these elements.

Earth Element

Din | ดิน

The most important thing to know about any element is the experience of that element. The experience of Earth is solidity, and therefore all things that we experience as solid, have excited Earth element. The primary qualities of Earth element are that it is hard, stable, and heavy, just like a boulder or a mountain. Earth constitutes all that is hard, solid, tangible, and has mass. It has form and the quality of being still. It is the heaviest of the elements, making it slow and dense. Earth is also considered to be moist, sweet, bulky, and rough, as well as dull, dense, gross, and not slimy. Think of a block of clay, how heavy and moist and scratchy it is. This is the Element earth. It is the function of Earth to provide resistance and support, like the walls of a building, a skeleton, a riverbed, or a cup.

Within the body, Earth dominates all that has mass, such as the bones, the organs,[38] the skin, and the nails. Earth is considered to be the container in which all the other elements reside. It gives structure and holds the body upright. It is the actual machinery that is functioning within the body. Earth is associated with the sense of smell (because it is earth particulates that contain scent), and the nose, as well as the expelling of waste, and the colon. Earth has a close relationship with Water (*Nam*), as they are the two heaviest elements and Earth needs Water to lubricate and bind it together. Without water, earth crumbles.

Traditionally there are twenty body parts associated with the Earth element in Thai medicine.[39] They are shown in the table below, and, like the qualities, are meant to be learned and memorized in the order presented. The list of body parts associated with Earth does not list every possible body part. The main reason for this is that many organs are considered part of a system. For example, the bladder is an extension of the kidneys, and the pancreas is seen as an extension of the liver. We can see this in the semantics of Thai anatomy. The Thai word for liver is *dtap*, and the Thai word for pancreas is *dtap awn* (ตับอ่อน), meaning "soft liver."

Another reason that there are twenty body parts associated with Earth is, because in Buddhism the number twenty has a sympathetic/magical significance with Earth element. This is taken into account in medical practices. For example, when treating Earth Traditional Thai Medicine practitioners might use a formula with twenty ingredients; or perhaps when working with the herb that is associated with Earth they will use twenty parts of that herb. A meditation on the Earth might be done every day for twenty days, or a chant might be chanted twenty times. Each of the elements has its own number association.

---

38 When talking about the organs in relation to Earth element, we are talking about the physical structure of the organ, not the function.

39 Lanna medicine recognizes 21.

Earth *Din* | ดิน		Earth Parts of the Body *Twenty Components*
Experience	Solidity	1. Hair on the head
Function	Provides resistance and support	2. Hair on the body (beard,eyebrows, armpit hair etc.)
Primary qualities	Hard, stable, heavy	
Other Qualities (not necessarily in trad. texts, but understood by practitioners)	Heavy • Stable • Dull • Dense • Gross • Non-Slimy (not wet) • Moist • Sweet • Bulky • Rough	3. Nails 4. Teeth
Temperature	Neither hot nor cold (sù-kŭm สุขุม)	5. Skin
Season	Between seasons, or winter	6. Muscles
Zodiac (vedic)	Taurus, Virgo, Capricorn	7. Tendons, Ligaments, Blood Vessels and Nerves (collectively known as *Sên*)
Number	Twenty	
Shape	Square	
Color	Yellow	8. Bone
Direction	South	9. Marrow

Look to the experience, the function and the qualities of Earth. All things that you encounter as being heavy, or providing structure and support, are demonstrating their Earth element, and all things that you encounter as being solid, are demonstrating their Earth element. This can be in degrees.

A somewhat malleable plastic cup, has solidity, and provides support for the drink within; here we can see the Earth element. A clay cup is more solid, less malleable, and therefore displaying the Earth element of its makeup more than the plastic cup. Yet we can see Earth in both. We can also see Earth in the nature of things such as a solid, dependable person who you know you can lean on for support.

10. Kidneys

11. Heart

12. Liver

13. Fascia

14. Spleen

15. Lungs

16. Large intestine

17. Small intestine

18. Stomach

19. Feces

20. Brain and Nervous system (counted as one)

Water Element
Nám | น้ำ

Water, like Earth, is a tangible element in the body that we can easily experience and understand. The experience of Water is fluidity, so everything that we encounter that has a fluid nature has excited Water element. On a physical level, it is literally the fluids within us, the blood sweat and tears of us. Water brings cohesion to our bodies, binding and sticking everything together. This can be understood when we think of how two droplets of water will stick together. It is what makes us supple and moist. Without water, earth would make everything too solid; we would be hard and crumbly. Water is the glue that holds us together. It allows for permeation and keeps us "well oiled." It is important to remember that the Water element in oceans and rivers, sap, and fruit juices embodies the same qualities of the water that is the blood, saliva, and synovial fluids within us. We are made of the same elements as everything around us.

Water has the primary qualities of being moist, fluid, and soft. It is also cold, heavy, sweet, dull, unctuous (oily), soft, and slimy. When most people think of water they think of a clear non-viscous liquid, so to understand how water can be unctuous and slimy you must understand that all liquid substances fall into this category, including sap, mucous, and blood. Because we need moisture in our mouths in order to taste, this is the sense that Water element is associated with, and the mouth is its sense organ.

The number twelve is associated with Water, with the twelve bodily fluids; like the number twenty associated with Earth, it comes into play in how medicine is created in connection to Water imbalances. The twelve body parts associated with Water, and the twenty body parts associated with Earth make up the thirty-two components of the physical body: twenty solid, twelve fluid. These are the actual tangible substances which we can touch, see and smell.

Of course, we have more than thirty-two body parts, so it is important to realize that numbers do not always stand for an exact quantity in Eastern sciences. For example, the number 108 is referred to in many Eastern texts. This number is sometimes representative of the actual quantity of 108, but more often than not it is representative of a nonspecific large amount. In this reference to the body parts, the thirty-two most important body parts are counted, but it is acknowledged that there are more.

Water Nám | น้ำ		Water Parts of the Body Twelve Components
Experience	Aqueous-ness (liquidity)	1. Bile Bile is divided into two categories: bound and unbound. Bound bile resides within the gallbladder while unbound bile resides outside the gallbladder
Function	Provides cohesion and fluidity	
Primary qualities	Moist, fluid, soft	
Other Qualities (not necessarily in trad. texts)	Cold • Heavy • Dull • Unctuous (oily) • Soft • Slimy • Sweet	
Temperature	Cold	2. Mucous Mucous is divided into three categories: Neck and head, chest, and below the naval. This is not inclusive of mucous specific to the nose and throat, which is listed separately.
Season	Winter/Spring	
Zodiac	Cancer, Scorpio, Pisces	
Number	12	
Shape	Circle	3. Pus
Color	White	4. Blood
Direction	East	5. Sweat

Look to the experience, the function, and the qualities of Water. All things that you encounter as having liquidity, are demonstrating their Water element, just as all things that you encounter as binding things together are demonstrating their Water element. This could be the glue that binds the parts of a wooden chair, or the nature of a team captain with a talent for creating unity in the team.

    Water also presents itself with sweetness, be it a flavor or a personality. When you notice these things, know that you are noticing the Water element . Water can also present as heavy. Heavy can confuse a bit as Earth is heavy as well. With practice, you will distinguish between the two.

6. Fat

7. Tears

8. Oil
Includes lymph

9. Saliva

10. Mucous of the Nose and Throat

11. Synovial Fluid

12. Urine

Fire Element

Fai | ไฟ

The experience of Fire is heat, and so all warmth and lack of warmth is related to Fire element. The primary qualities of Fire are that it is bright, reactive, and sharp. Fire is also dry, rough, light, unctuous (oily), mobile, hot, and non-slimy.

Because our eyes take in light, it is associated with the sense of sight, and the eyes are its sense organ. Fire is also associated with the urge to move and the number four. Just as Earth has twenty component parts in the body, and Water has twelve, Fire has four[40]: the Fire that provides warmth for the body, the Fire that causes aging and decay,[41] the Fire that causes emotion and fever, and the Fire of digestion. Digestion is Fire's most important, or primary job; however, Fire is also associated with other important aspects such as willpower, passion, motivation, and fortitude.

While Earth and Water are the tangible physical elements of the body, Fire is more of a metabolic process, a function rather than a physical component. Fire cannot be touched like Water and Earth can, but along with Wind it brings life to those two elements. Fire is the impetus for movement; it heats our body and preserves it. Fire provides warmth, body heat, and circulation. It also provides passion, willpower, an ability to see clearly, anger, and articulation of ideas. Fire equates to metabolism, digestion, and heat and is associated with hormones. Fire is what gives us the energy to change, mature, transform, and have impetus.

---

40 In Lanna medicine, Fire has six component parts: 1. Fire that heats the body and gives us energy; 2. Fire of digestion; 3. Fire of emotion and impetus; 4. Fire of aging and decay; 5. Fire that maintains balance with the thirty-two constituent parts; and 6. Fire that connects consciousness to the body.

41 Think of how the sun (fire) transforms a sour young plum into a delicious sweet fruit.

Fire *Fai* | ไฟ		Fire Parts of the Body *Four Components*
Experience	Heat	1. Fire that provides warmth for the body
Function	Provides transformation and ripening	
		2. Fire that causes emotion and fever
Primary qualities	Bright, reactive, sharp	
Other Qualities (learn in order)	Sharp • Dry • Rough • Light • Unctuous (oily) • Mobile • Non-slimy • Hot	3. Fire that causes aging and decay (ripening)
		4. Fire that digests food
Temperature	Hot	
Season	Summer	
Zodiac	Aries, Leo, Sagittarius	
Number	Four	
Shape	Triangle	
Color	Red	
Direction	West	

Look to the experience, function and qualities of Fire. All things that you encounter as being hot, are demonstrating their Fire element. This is inclusive of temperature and personality (as seen in the idiom "hot headed". Keep in mind that all things have all elements, such that even a frozen lake contains Fire, but the Fire element is in a weakened state. If it did not contain Fire, it would not warm and melt with the arrival of spring activating the Fire within.

Fire is also encountered as reactive, and so anything that you experience as such is demonstrating its Fire element. We also see Fire in all transformation, ripening and decay, from the fruit bud that transforms into fruit and ripens on the tree, and eventually decays, to ideas that form and mature and change over time.

Wind Element

Lom | ลม

First, semantics. The word *lom* (ลม) is often mistakenly translated as "air" in English language texts on Thai medicine. However, the correct translation of *lom* is "wind." The distinction is important, as Wind element is movement. While air can be stagnant, wind cannot. Thai, like English, has a separate word for air: *aa-gàat* (อากาศ), and one should not be substituted for the other as it will lead to confusion when understanding Thai medicine. It is extremely important to realize that every single movement we make, be it breathing, speaking, running, hiccuping, or shivering, is connected to Wind element. The relationship of movement and Wind element is that they are one and the same, and whether you use the Thai word *Lom* or stick to the English word Wind, in the context of traditional medicine these words should be synonymous with "movement," as movement is the experience of Wind element. The sooner this is truly grasped, the sooner you will understand this element, as well as many factors of Thai healing arts.

In addition to mobility, the other primary qualities of Wind element are that it is light (not heavy) and dry. Additionally Wind has the qualities of being cool, rough, un-unctuous, subtle, and non-slimy. By rough what is meant is that Wind has an abrasive quality to it. It can wear things down, or be cutting. When we speak of Wind as being movement, we acknowledge the sameness of the wind that blows through the branches of the trees dancing the leaves, as the wind that activates our legs to run and our thoughts to progress from one to the next.

Wind, like Fire, is more of a metabolic process than a tangible element in the body. Wind is what animates us, gives life to form. If Earth and Water are the anatomy of us, then Fire and Wind are the physiology of us. While Fire is the impetus for movement, Wind is responsible for the movement itself. From the movement of walking or turning the pages of a book to the movement of digestion and from the motion of blood circulating through our arteries and veins to the motion of our thoughts circulating through our minds, it is Wind that creates the movement.

Wind is the lightest of the elements mentioned thus far and is therefore the element that is most easily thrown out of balance or disturbed. For this reason, and because Wind is what animates the other elements, it is often one of the most important elements to look at when making elemental diagnosis. Just about all traditional medicine systems speak of Wind element as being a major disease-causing factor.

Wind is associated with the sense of touch (think of wind brushing against your skin) and, if using Thai Five Element theory, hearing (wind carries sound to our ears). Due to this the skin and ears are the sense organs of Wind.

Wind falls into two categories: gross and subtle. Gross forms of Wind make up all the tangible physical motions, from running to the circulation of blood. The movement of food traveling through the digestive tract, the movement of a baby being born, the movement of writing, defecating, and smiling—all of these are gross forms of Wind. The subtle Wind elements make up all of the intangible movements, such as the motion of thoughts, emotions, ideas, remembering, urges, habits, and our sense of self. Bodywork mostly focuses on the gross forms of Wind element, of which there are six primary forms[42] that require discussion at this level of training; six is the number association with Wind.

1. Ascending Wind

This Wind moves from the feet or the abdomen (depending on what texts/teachers the information comes from) to the top of the head and works in conjunction with, or paired with, the descending Wind. Ascending Wind relates to all upward motion, such as blood moving up the body, vomiting, belching, voice, hiccups, upward circulation, and receptive (afferent) nerve impulses to the spine and brain.

2. Descending Wind

This Wind moves from the top of the head to the feet, or the abdomen (depending on which texts/teachers the information comes from) and represents all descending movement in the body. This includes such movements as gas, downward arterial flow, urination, childbirth, ejaculation, and menstruation. This Wind is connected to the efferent (motor) neural pathways carrying impulses away from the central nervous system. Descending Wind must work in conjunction with Ascending Wind.

3. Wind Within the Digestive Tract

This Wind helps to push food down the digestive tract. Rumblings in the digestive system and gas from foods fermenting within us are examples of imbalances of this Wind; however, it should be noted that this Wind is often created from the external, from Wind that is swallowed while eating and talking. This swallowed Wind is necessary for expansion within the digestive tract; however, too much of it can be problematic. Thai medicine teaches that the ideal balance of substances taken into the digestive tract are two parts food, one part water, and one part wind. The Wind element inside the digestive tract also separates waste food from nutrient food.

4. Wind in the Abdomen, but Outside the Digestive Tract

This Wind is responsible for movement such as peristalsis and smooth muscle contraction, as well as other mechanical functions of the organs, such as excretion of gallbladder fluids, active kidney, spleen and liver function, heart contraction, and so on. This Wind is paired with the Wind within the digestive tract.

5. Wind that Circulates to all Parts of the Body, Including the Extremities

This Wind is primarily related to the circulation of blood throughout the body, but it is also connected to nervous impulses and motor control of muscles. It moves the five branches of the body, which are made up of the four extremities and the head. This Wind, more than any other, is affected by bodywork. This is because this wind relates to movement throughout the body,

---

42 Lanna medicine uses seven Winds.

and one of the primary functions of bodywork is to free up blockages such that there is free movement of everything, from blood to ideas.

6. *Wind of Respiration*

This Wind is related to the external Wind that is inhaled into the body, processed by the heart, and circulated through the body. It descends, ascends, and moves throughout the body. This Wind can be paired with the Wind that circulates to all parts of the body, including the extremities. The Wind of respiration is special because it is the one Wind that we can control.

In subcategories of these six winds, all human movements have their own Wind. For instance, the Wind that turns the unborn baby into the head-down position before birth is a specific Wind, and the Wind that pushes the baby out into the world is a specific Wind, and every sense organ has a gross Wind that makes it function (although a subtle Wind carries the knowledge of the sense to consciousness). Tradition holds that there are 108 Winds in the body; however, this number is likely more symbolic than exact.

Wind *Lom* | ลม		Wind Parts of the Body *Six Components*
Experience	Movement	1. Ascending Wind that moves from the feet to the head
Function	Provides growth and vibration	
Primary qualities	Light, mobile, dry	2. Descending Wind that moves from the head to the feet
Other Qualities (learn in order)	Light • Cool • Rough • Ununctuous • Subtle • Non-Slimy	3. Wind inside the digestive tract
Temperature	Cool	4. Wind outside the digestive tract but inside the abdomen
Zodiac	Gemini, Libra, Aquarius	
Number	Six	5. Wind the circulates throughout the body
Shape	Crescent	
Color	Green	6. Wind of respiration
Direction	North	
Look to the experience, function and qualities of Wind. All things that you encounter as having or being in motion are demonstrating their Wind element. This is inclusive of the movement of growth, the movement of thoughts, and the movement of a shiver through the body or a car on a racetrack. You are also encountering the Wind element when you notice the quality of anything being dry, very light, or the temperature as cool.		

Space Element

Aa-gàat tâat | อากาศธาตุ

Space is by far the easiest element to misunderstand or overlook, and yet on many levels is a very important element. Space is, well, space. It is emptiness; it is the atmosphere; it is the blackness of outer space; it is the empty places within our body; it is the space between atoms. Without the Space element nothing else would exist. The nature of space is to be empty and expansive, so when working with the Space element within us these are the qualities we look for. Are the places in the body that should have space in them free? Is there space for things to move and grow? How about our minds? Is there spaciousness, or are our minds full of thoughts and feelings and ideas? Maintaining the Space element in our lives/minds/bodies is of utmost importance for maintaining our health—mental, spiritual, and physical.

Despite all of this, the Space element is not always considered in Traditional Thai Medicine. It depends on which foundational texts are being referenced, who the doctor is, perhaps even what day it is. It is not that the Space element isn't acknowledged as important, but rather is: a) grouped with Wind; b) considered so all-pervasive as to not require specific notice; and c) Space is so very subtle, it just isn't a very tangible element.

Some people view the Space element from the Buddhist perspective, which says that all things are within the void, or Space. Another way to consider this is to say that at the most minute level, all things are really just made up of the Space element; there is a sort of finality and infinity to it. We see this concept in quantum physics when looking at the dominance of nothing. Others look at Space as that which is free or empty in the body. In most cases, these are the "open organs"—organs such as the stomach, the large intestines, the lungs, and the bladder, that connect to the external world.

In the Western science of quantum physics, space is acknowledged as the absence of matter, and it is said that there is more nothing than something, not only in outer space but also in our direct environment, with atoms being 99.99 percent empty space. There are quantum physics theories regarding the origins of the universe stemming from the vacuum of nothingness. In ancient Wiccan philosophy, space is said to be the beginning and ending, the all and the nothing. Likewise in Ayurvedic medicine, space is considered the beginning and end of all manifestation. In traditional Chinese medicine, space is not considered one of the five elements; however, the concept of Space is found in the Chinese philosophy of *Wuji*, or the emptiness from which all things come. The idea of emptiness, and emptiness being an originating factor, is universal in both new and ancient philosophies, but how it is applied in medicine differs from one culture to another.

If we look at the elements listed thus far, we can see that they are listed from heaviest or densest (Earth) to lightest (Wind, then Space). You will notice that Wind and Space share many qualities, but they are not the same. Space has no temperature association. It is smooth, without resistance, light, and expansive. In terms of Traditional Thai Medicine, the Space element has two primary associations: with the orifices of the body and with the mind.

Association with the Orifices of the Body

As pertains to the orifices of the body, the Space element involves the interaction of the environment outside the body with the environment inside the body. The places of exchange, or contact between the internal and the external, or the orifices:

- The eyes (2)
- The ears (2)
- The nostrils (2)
- The mouth (1)
- The anus (1)
- The urethra (1)
- The vagina (1)

Added up, we see that there are ten orifices (nine in men), so this number is associated with the Space element and its relation to the body. In addition to the orifices, there is an exchange between the internal and the external that occurs at the level of the skin and the blood that must also be taken into account when working with this Space association. All of the places where the external environment enters the internal, and vice versa, are places that create an equilibrium between the outer and inner worlds. When we are considering environmental factors in disease, it's always necessary to address these areas, and therefore this element. Furthermore, the sensory input we receive from these locations helps to form our body's energy and to shape the mind. If, for example, our ears are exposed to loud or unpleasant sounds, or our mouth encounters noxious-tasting food, this may cause a disharmony in the body.

In bodywork, the relationship with the Space element is about making sure there is Space in the body where it needs to be, and therefore goes beyond the orifices. In this context, we consider Space between muscles, Space between ligaments, the removal of adhesions, and the separation of bound tissues.

Blood

Lêuat | เลือด, *or the more medical term Loh-hìt* | โลหิต

Blood encompasses the three main elements in a very special way and is considered the essence of our existence. It is one of the most important aspects of the body, and is sometimes considered to be a separate element unto itself, as it is comprised of Water, Fire, and Wind. The motion of blood is Wind, its heat is Fire, and its fluidity is Water. Blood must be considered in any condition or imbalance, with each of its elemental aspects being cared for. The fluidity (Water aspect) is dependent upon the blood being clean, without toxins or excess fatty matter. The flow and circulation (Wind aspect) of blood must be smooth and balanced, and the temperature (Fire aspect) of blood must be balanced and harmonized to the body's health needs. Traditional Thai Medicine states that if you can heal the blood, you can heal the entire person. Blood is what nourishes and connects the body, and is the essence of humans.

Bringing it Together

The elements are the primary building blocks of all matter, and all things, living and nonliving, are made of all the elements in various levels of excitement. We can see that the elements, in any form, are constantly interacting with one another, both in external nature and within our own bodies. The dynamic three elements of Water, Fire, and Wind constantly play with each other.

Understanding how the elements relate to and differentiate from one another will guide you to deeper knowledge of the body and the world. Space, the lightest element, cannot be felt, seen, tasted, or smelled, but it can be heard. Wind, the next lightest element, is the most easily distorted, the fastest to change. Wind can be heard and felt but cannot be seen, tasted, or smelled. Fire is slightly heavier than Wind, but it is still light. It can change easily but not quite as easily as Wind. Fire can be heard, felt, and seen but cannot be tasted or smelled. Water is heavy and does not change easily. Water can be heard, felt, seen, and tasted but not smelled. Earth is the heaviest element, the hardest to change. Earth can be heard, felt, seen, tasted, and smelled. Wind, Fire, and Water are contained by Earth, and they all occupy Space.

Element theory is essential to Traditional Thai Medicine, just as atoms and molecules are essential to Western medicine and yin and yang are essential to traditional Chinese medicine. In Traditional Thai Medicine, everything begins and ends with the elements. The elements each exist in the body and have their specific jobs to do. If one of these elements becomes unbalanced you may not notice, but the one unbalanced element will lead to others being unbalanced until the body becomes ill. The concepts presented in this section will resound throughout the rest of this book, so the reader is encouraged to study this section well before moving on.

Core Elemental Constitution

When we look at a person as a whole, we find that each individual has a core elemental constitution, meaning that some people are more innately fiery, some are more innately windy, and some are more innately watery. Our core elemental constitution affects everything from physique to disease propensity to character traits. A person's core elemental constitution can be one element, or a combination of two, or in some cases even three elements in equal proportion (although the latter is rare).

If more than one element exists strongly in someone but not in equal measure, the element that is slightly less is considered a secondary core constitution. For example, a person's core elemental constitution may be equally Fire and Wind, or be predominantly Fire, but have Wind coming in as a close secondary element in that person's constitutional makeup. The first scenario can be worded with either element stated first, but in the latter scenario the person's elemental constitution would be termed "Fire/Wind."

A person's elemental constitution is determined by the time of conception (season and astrological factors), parents, type of pregnancy (including what foods the mother eats and where she lives), and time of day of birth. Once you are born, you already have a core elemental constitution, but for approximately the first six years of life your constitution can be changed by life habits and environment. Once you are about six years old, it cannot change anymore. Elemental constitution stays the same throughout a person's life; however, it is possible (and common) for people to have an elemental imbalance at any given moment that is different from their core elemental constitution. So a person with a Water constitution, for example, can have a Wind imbalance of amplified Wind, and they will manifest Wind-related problems. Understanding the imbalance is much more imperative to a healing arts practitioner than understanding the core constitution, but ideally it's good to know both.

> *Core elemental constitution is the elemental baseline for an individual — the element or elements that dominate in the absence of an imbalance. The difference between the core elemental constitution and an elemental imbalance is that the core elemental constitution is what we are born with and the imbalance is what we make.*

A person with a Water constitution is naturally more watery than a person with a Fire constitution, and a person with a Wind constitution is naturally more windy than either the Fire or the Water person. The core elemental constitution is not a cause for concern and does not require treatment; however, knowing a person's core elemental constitution brings greater understanding of the extent of imbalance.

Imagine if everyone had the potential to have very different normal body temperatures instead of the average 98.6º (F), 37º (C). Before a doctor could assess whether their patient had a fever, he or she would have to first find out what the patient's normal body temperature was. Sometimes, in order to know if someone has say, a Wind imbalance, one must first know what the patient's core elemental constitution is. An element far out of balance shows itself as clearly not healthy, but knowing the core elemental constitution will help in determining just how far out of balance it is and is useful when an element is only slightly unbalanced.

For example, two people displaying the exact same agitated Wind symptoms, but one with Water as their core elemental constitution and the other with Wind as their core elemental constitution, are displaying two very different levels of imbalance. For this reason, it is ideal to get to know people when they are relatively healthy and the core elemental constitution can be more easily determined. This ideal is not always possible, however, so it is important to study the elements, meditate on them, and watch for them in as many people as possible in order to start to get a sense of indicators of the core elemental constitution versus indicators of imbalance.

Core elemental constitution is not fixed in early childhood and, although it's rare, it can change up until about age six, due to such factors as environment and diet. As I mentioned earlier, once a person's elemental constitution is fixed, it remains for life and does not change. When learning about core elemental constitutions, it is important to remember that the lists of characteristics given are generalizations based on frequently found qualities, but everyone will not present in the same way. Dark hair, for example, is a common characteristic with Wind constitution, but it is certainly possible for a Wind constitution person to present with blond hair. When trying to decipher a person's elemental constitution one looks at the preponderance of characteristics and usually combines this evidence with other diagnostic tools that will be discussed later in this book.

Again, please keep in mind as we look at how core constitutions present that the core elemental constitution is not unto itself a problem and doesn't need to be "treated." What we are looking at in the following descriptions is a normal and balanced state for different core elemental constitutions, and it is only imbalances (which we will get to in a bit) that need to be treated. In the absence of an imbalance, we look to the core elemental constitution to see how best to maintain good health.

Earth as a Core Elemental Constitution

PHYSICAL CHARACTERISTICS: The part Earth plays in a person's elemental makeup will contribute to them having a large frame, being big boned, big eyed, strong and muscular, or heavy set, with a deep resonant voice. They will usually have many characteristics also found in people with a Water constitution, such as thick hair and large eyes, but they will have more of a solidity to them, a squareness of shape, and significantly bigger skeletal frames.

MENTAL CHARACTERISTICS: When looking for Earth qualities in a person think of farmers, think of terms like "salt of the earth" or "grounded." These are people potentially with a lot of Earth element. People with Earth as a core elemental constitution tend to like hearth and home and eschew adventure and travel. They have a steadiness of mind and may be slow to change. People with a lot of Earth element usually to have good perspective and a compassionate balanced nature. Be careful of the idea that anyone who likes to walk barefoot, bakes pies from scratch, and dries their own mint tea is "earthy" and therefore must have be Earth constitution. The association with Earth, and a nature-loving character type, or the stereotype of a "hippie," is not the same as having Earth core elemental constitution.

Water as Core Elemental Constitution

PHYSICAL CHARACTERISTICS: People with Water core elemental constitution tend to have a balanced and well-shaped or larger, more corpulent figure and a healthy complexion. They are known to often have large "sweet" eyes with thick lashes. They generally have full, thick, dark hair and a clear, soft, melodious voice. Their skin tone is usually full, soft, and hydrated, like a child's. They have a steady stride and a balanced gait. Their face structure is usually wider toward the mouth and chin. Water-dominant people often have a high tolerance for hunger and both heat and cold. While Water constitution people can tend toward being overweight, in general they are known for their beauty.[43] Water-constitutions often have slow digestion and are easily injured and slow to heal. Because Water is heavy and slow, energy will have to work harder to move through the channels of the body, so Watery people tend to hold onto toxins and get sick more easily.

MENTAL CHARACTERISTICS: People with a Water core elemental constitution tend to be easy-going and flexible, with an inner sweetness. They are often intuitive and drawn to healing or creative arts, and are generally kind. They think a lot but are not good at decision-making, preferring either consciously or subconsciously to allow others to guide their choices. They have malleable minds and so are easily led. They can be introspective and are at risk of depres-

---

43 While certain Water characteristics, such as large eyes, thick lashes, and full lips, are still considered beautiful, modern-day beauty standards lean more toward athletic Fire bodies, or extra-thin Wind bodies. The concepts presented here stem from times long ago, and these sorts of standards can change.

sion. Water-dominant people can be slow learners. As Water is a heavy element, thoughts and new ideas do not process quickly through it, but once something is learned, they tend to remember it. If they suffer from fear and anxiety, it comes from a lack of understanding. Because Water is the glue, they are often the one who "holds things together." Water-dominant people can become stuck on thoughts and ideas, having a difficult time seeing other points of view. Water is emotional, especially with emotions such as sadness, nostalgia, yearning, happiness, fullness, and emptiness. Watery people are more prone to tears than other elemental constitutions. Water constitution often has a low sex drive, moderate sweat, and moderate scent. Water, Fire, and Wind each have a specific mental defect associated with them, and Water's mental defect is ignorance.

AGE: Regardless of our core elemental constitution, when we are very young, Water is a dominant element. You can see it in the plump, hydrated skin tone of babies and children, their big sweet eyes, and in their tendency toward mucousy noses, strong emotions, and easy tearfulness. Small children have rapidly growing changing bodies, and Water is an element of becoming, creation. Children are intuitive and receptive—characteristics of Water. The element of Water is particularly strong from birth until around age eight. Then from eight to sixteen years of age, Water is still very present but waning, as Fire is increasing.

Fire as a Core Elemental Constitution

PHYSICAL CHARACTERISTICS: Fiery people tend to have reddish to tan complexions, and cliché as it may seem, red headed people invariably have Fire core elemental constitution. People with Fire as a primary element are generally of average build, with clear sharp eyes. They have soft hair, including facial hair, and are prone to wrinkles, loose joints, and early graying. Fire causes strong-smelling urine, sweat, and breath because of the degree to which it is constantly breaking down nutrients. Fire constitution people generally have strong digestion as well as a strong athletic build.

MENTAL CHARACTERISTICS: People with Fire core elemental constitution tend to be very intelligent, catching on quickly and able to easily articulate thoughts and get to the point. They have a tendency toward leadership and instruction, and they make good speakers. They are also very driven, with Fire creating a tendency toward ideas and change, however they can lean toward selfishness. Fire constitution people are often short-tempered and may be aggressive or bully others, either physically, emotionally, or mentally (consciously or unconsciously). They have a strong sense of self, strong willpower, and a strong sex drive. Fire's mental defect association is aversion.

AGE: Regardless of what a person's core elemental constitution is, Fire begins to come in as a strong element around age eight, and increases until it becomes the dominant element from our mid teens into our early thirties. This is a time of passions, anger, intensity, sexuality, and often driven productivity. We can see in teenagers outward signs of Fire manifesting in acne, sweat, and strong emotions, especially anger and passion. Fire is central from approximately age sixteen until around age thirty-two. This does not mean that it becomes the core elemental constitution, just that in everyone, this is an extra fiery time. From age thirty-two until age sixty-four, Fire is waning and Wind is increasing.

Wind as a Core Elemental Constitution

PHYSICAL CHARACTERISTICS: People with Wind core elemental constitution tend to be either very tall or very short, with light small bodies regardless of height. They lean toward small skeletal structure, being thin, and having small eyes and dark coloring. Their skin tends to be dry, and their faces are wider toward the forehead and eyes. They have smaller eyes, a dark complexion, and difficulty staying warm.

MENTAL CHARACTERISTICS: Windy people are often very academically intelligent, grasping new ideas quickly. However, their thoughts and communication can be erratic and jump from one subject to the next without going into depth in any one area. The classic description of "flighty" may be applied to them. They are often mathematical, good at computer work, and artistic. Windy people tend to have lots of ideas but do not always have the focus to carry them through. They are often anxious, nervous, chaotic, fast-paced, and creative, and they are easily overstimulated. Because spirits are extremely windy, people with a predominance of Wind may connect to them easily (for better or worse). Wind's mental defect association is attachment.

AGE: Around age thirty-two, the Wind element begins to increase regardless of what element a person's core elemental constitution is. This increase in Wind continues for the rest of our lives, becoming strongest after age sixty-four. We can see this in elderly people who have become overly anxious, their skin dry and brittle, their nights insomniac (that is, restless).

Sên Theory | เส้น

Let's begin our exploration by first looking at the Thai word *sên*.[44] It has many meanings, and by listing a handful of them we begin to form an umbrella understanding of the word. For "*sên*" can mean a route, a street, a noodle, a hair, an equator, a nerve, a vein, a tendon, a path, a line or a string. Getting it? For our intentions, my favorite explanation is that a *sên* is "a physical pathway by which movement occurs in the body." I want to say that last part once more, because I think it is important:

> **A *sên* is a physical pathway by which movement occurs in the body.**

Okay, that feels good. Now I'll unpack it.

Let's start by spending a moment looking at what *sên* are not. They are not the same as Chinese meridians. They are an entirely different system, and the *sên* lines do not correspond to organs or elements in the same way they do in traditional Chinese medicine. They do not follow the same pathways, are not made of the same substances, and while they can distally refer, they are not reflexive, as with Chinese meridians. *Sên* are also not mystical hollow tubes in the body through which a metaphysical force invisibly blows. Sên are not the same as yogic *nāḍī,* but they are similar to Ayurvedic *nādi.*

It is very important to understand *sên* within their own system of Traditional Thai Medicine. It does not work to intermix medical theory, even when some overlapping ideas exist. For those who have studied Chinese and/or Indian medical systems, it is necessary to keep them separate. They are wonderful and complicated systems in their own right, but they do not have an application here.

For the most part, *sên* are tangible structures. Most of the *sên* that we work with in the body are tendons, ligaments, veins, nerves, and arteries. They also sometimes refer to muscular and fascial pathways. If you look at the twenty body parts made of Earth element you will see many of these structures listed as a group making up the seventh body part (tendons/ligaments/vessels/nerves). As you know by now, it is the parts of us that are most palpable, visible, and measurable that are made of Earth element. So really the *sên* are made of the Earth element. They are also the pathways of the substances that we cannot so easily see, such as hormones and electrical impulses (these are known as the invisible *sên,* but I'll get to that in a moment). Because of the common misconception that *sên* are metaphysical, invisible, or purely spiritual lines, this all takes a bit of extra explanation.

It is frequently understood that *sên* are routes by which Wind flows through the body. This is mostly true; however, it is an explanation that leads to quite a lot of confusion, as people

---

44 Notice that I do not call them "*sên* lines." This is because to do so is redundant if you know the meaning of the word *sên.* It's a bit like saying "Thank you" every time you use the Spanish word *gracias,* which would mean "Thank you, thank you." Saying "*sên* line" is like saying "line line." Also, I have another purpose for the word line in this book.

imagine invisible tubes with invisible breezes blowing through them, and overlay terms from other systems such as *qi* (*chi*), *prāna*, or the ever tricky word "energy."[45] So hold in mind that we are dealing with earthy, tangible structures.

Now, go back to the section in this chapter on Elements. Read about the Wind element. It says that Wind is all movement, right? So when we talk about Wind in the *sên*, what is meant is that these channels are—you know where I'm going here, yes?—pathways by which movement occurs in the body. Real movement, in real pathways. The flow of blood, muscular contraction, the jumping of electrical impulses—these are all tangible, animating forces in our bodies. And in Thai physiology, all that movement is Wind. This combination of physical structures (Earth) and movement (Wind) makes the *sên* both physical and energetic. In this context, the word "energy" is used to mean a "moving force."

The Wind element is incredibly important in Traditional Thai Medicine. When dealing with the *sên*, the job of the bodyworker is to manipulate the Wind element in order to free up the passageways. A Thai bodyworker doesn't think about releasing tight muscles so much as they think about freeing the Wind. It may result in the same work, but the outlook is important, for ultimately one of the primary goals of Thai bodywork is to allow for the smooth flow of Wind (movement) in the body.

To do this, to access and work with the *sên*, one often has to spend time on the tissue layer of the body, the fascia, and muscles, but they are not the end goal. You do not release a muscle for its own sake; you do it because in so doing you cause movement of the body to be unimpaired. You heal the flow of Wind. Beyond this, with Thai bodywork you can do things such as regulate Wind flow, smooth erratic Wind, build deficient Wind, and more.

As mentioned earlier, the Thai word for wind is *lom*. This word, like *sên*, can have many meanings. It can be the wind in the body, the wind outside, the wind of respiration, the wind of your thoughts; it can even refer to ghosts (which are quite windy). In this context, when we talk about *lom* in relation to the *sên*, we are talking about movement in the body. It is simply another word for Wind.

There are four divisions of *sên*:

MAJOR *SÊN*: These are the main arteries, nerves, lymph ducts, tendons, and ligaments.

MINOR *SÊN*: These are the smaller vessels that branch off from the Major *Sên*, such as smaller vascular pathways, neural offshoots, and smaller lymphatic vessels.

INVISIBLE *SÊN*: The invisible *sên* are made up of the connections and pathways of hormones, neurons, neurotransmitters, and enzymes; they are not visible to the naked eye. While bodywork may have an effect upon them, such as endorphin release, for the most part these *sên* are treated with herbs and diet, not external body therapies.

---

45 The word "energy" can be used to mean an electrical current, the force of a punch, how much vitality and strength you have at the moment, a vibe coming off someone, or the idea of sending invisible healing. Because of the lack of precision of meaning with this word, I do not use it often.

SUBTLE *SÊN*: These are the pathways of the subtle Winds. They are ethereal pathways, psychic pathways, and pathways of emotion and thought.

Tradition says that there are 72,000 *sên* in the body. This number is representative of the uncountable, the infinite. If you think of all the possible pathways of movement in the body—all the veins, arteries, neural pathways, lymphatic passages, tendons, ligaments, muscles, and interstitial fluid routes—it is easy to understand why.

Trenches/Lines

Usually when people learn Thai bodywork they are taught the *sên* as numbered lines on the body (for example, Inside Lower Leg Line 1, Outside Upper Arm Line 2, and so forth). These lines are most often spaces, or trenches, where you can easily access the deeper body. They are not the *sên* themselves, but many *sên* can be accessed through them. There is no Thai word for these lines, but terms such as trenches, lines or spaces work to describe them. These trenches are most often found in the spaces between major body structures, such as between bone and muscle or between two muscles.

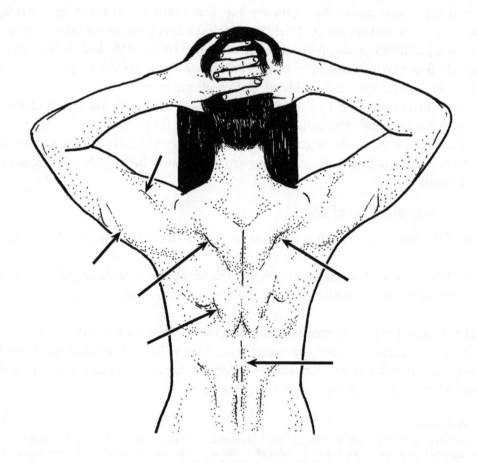

In a healthy body, if you press in these channels with your thumb, your thumb will sink deeper into the body than it will if you press directly on the muscles. It is a place that should allow for greater penetration. Because of this, veins, nerves, and other *sên* can be better accessed.

It must be understood that the concept of depth is relative to where you are on the body. For instance, the trenches found between the major muscles of the thigh are quite deep. In contrast, the trenches of the dorsal foot, have very little tissue around them, and therefore the distance a thumb can sink is greatly reduced. However, in relation to the amount of tissue, trenches do exist on the dorsal foot.

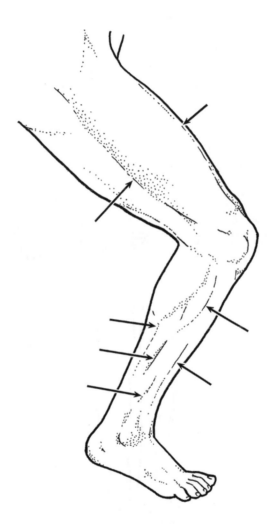

The diagrams on the following pages show many of the biggest and most commonly utilized trenches, but once you understand what the trenches are you won't need charts to show you. Simply follow the lines in the body, the places that border and outline bones, muscles, tendons, and ligaments.

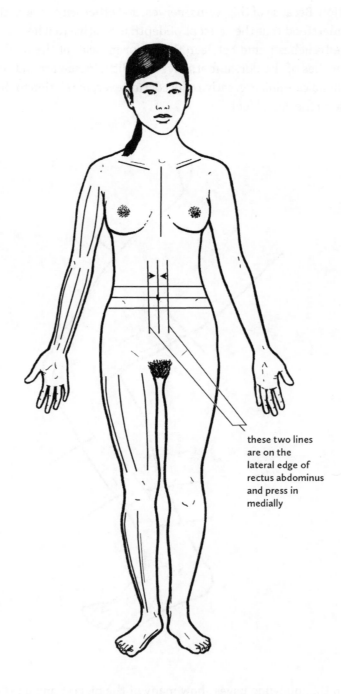

these two lines
are on the
lateral edge of
rectus abdominus
and press in
medially

Important Lines of the Anterior Body

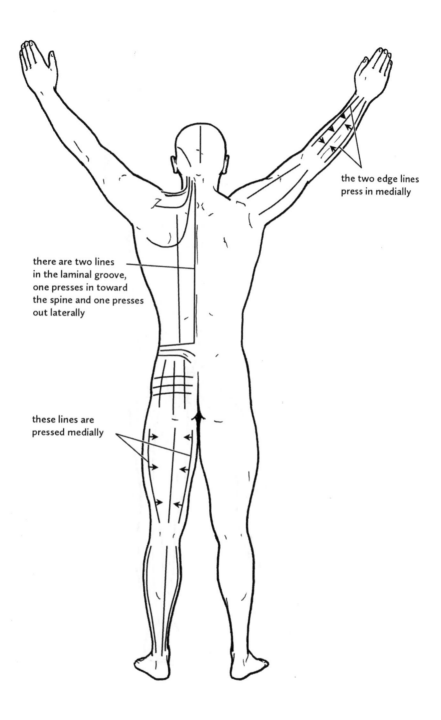

the two edge lines
press in medially

there are two lines
in the laminal groove,
one presses in toward
the spine and one presses
out laterally

these lines are
pressed medially

Important Lines of the Posterior Body

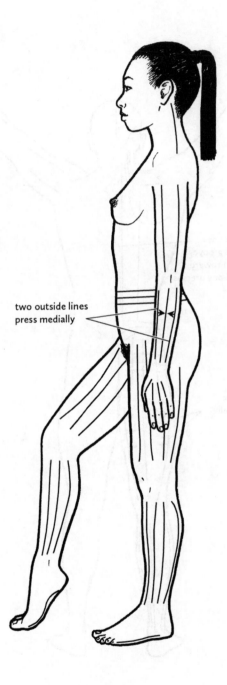

two outside lines
press medially

Important Lines Along the Side of the Body

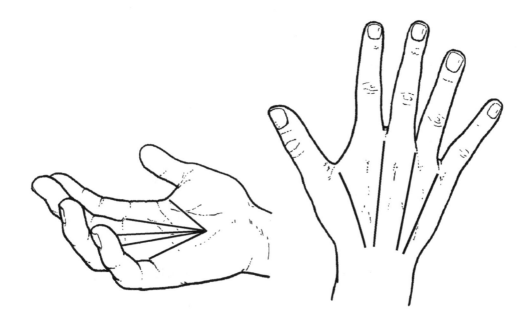

Important Lines of the Hands

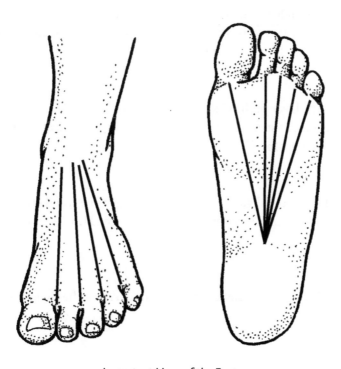

Important Lines of the Feet

Three Aspects

Another layer of Thai anatomy/physiology is the three aspects:[46] the physical aspect, the energetic aspect, and the consciousness aspect. It is important to understand that Traditional Thai Medicine does not separate these parts of self. The physical, the energetic, and consciousness are all mixed in a cosmic blender such that they cannot be dissected apart—to touch one is to touch all. For this reason, you cannot just do bodywork or just do "energy work." While I can write about them one at a time, in a list, it simply is not possible to separate out the pieces of our being in real life.

The physical aspect is that which makes up our physical, tangible body, so Earth and Water are the main elements that one thinks of in connection to it. The energetic aspect has Wind and Fire association and is that which animates us, brings us to life. The consciousness aspect is associated with karma, thoughts, and the mind, and the elements of Space and Consciousness.

Layers of the Physical Body

The physical body described above is made of five layers as follows:

Skin

This is the outermost layer of the body and is often the point of entry for disease-causing pathogens such as heat, cold, Wind, dampness, germs, and so on. The skin is an organ of both absorption and elimination, so while it can take on pathogens and toxins, it is also one of the ways that we release them. There are three layers of skin mentioned in Thai medical texts, which roughly correlate to the epidermis, dermis, and hypodermis.

Tissue

Just below the skin is the layer of the tissue made primarily of fascia, muscle, and fat. This layer easily takes on pathogens, as seen when a chill wind hitting the skin at night becomes a muscular crick in the neck by morning.

Sên

This layer refers to the tendons, ligaments, veins, nerves, arteries, and other pathways of movement. Because the *sên* are areas of movement, they can spread things from the tissue to the rest of the body.

Bone

The next layer of the body is the skeletal structure, underlying the tissue and channels.

---

46 The aspects are sometimes misinterpreted as chakras. Chakras are a uniquely Indian concept not found in Thai medicine.

Organs

Organs can be divided into two categories: open organs, those that have connection to the external world such as lungs, bladder and stomach, and closed organs, such as the heart, liver, and spleen, which do not connect to the external. In a disease progression that begins with skin, open organs are reached before closed organs.

This understanding of the five layers of the physical body is extremely important in bodywork. Bodyworkers generally reach to the layer of the channels, and sometimes to the bone and the organs. All bodyworkers deal with skin and tissue. Understanding the order in which these layers are accessed affects our choices in how we work. For example, a massage therapist must always warm up the skin layer of the body before addressing the tissue layer, and the channels, which are a major focus in Thai bodywork, often cannot be reached until the tissue layer has been released.

It is important to listen to each layer, to be aware when there is resistance, and not to force your way past an area that is not ready. The layers of the body also comes into play in herbal formulations for the body; if you were to make a balm for achy muscles, you would need to put in herbs that get past the skin layer. The concept of the layers of the physical body, while taking up only a small portion of the book here, will be mentioned over and over, and must be prominent in any bodyworker's awareness.

Kwăn | ขวัญ

Another part of Thai anatomy/physiology is *kwăn*. There is no English equivalent word to *Kwăn*, so I will ask you to accept that none of the words I will use here to explain are exactly right, but hopefully together they will form an idea that is close.

Kwăn is the life force, animating spirit, or life force essence of the components of the body. It is a concept that has its roots in pre-Buddhist Animism and is found throughout Southeast Asia, the Himalayas, and China.[47] *Kwăn* are not reincarnating sorts of spirits, or the spirit that becomes a ghost or goes to heaven, but rather a life force spirit for each component of your current life body. When you die, the elements of your body return to pure element (think of the body decomposing into Earth and your last breath exhaling into the Winds of the world). Likewise, the *kwăn* simply dissolves into pure spirit. In Thailand, it is believed that every part of your body has its own individual *kwăn*. Your heart has the heart *kwăn*, your liver has the liver *kwăn*, your kidneys have kidney *kwăn*, and so on.

Kwăn maintain the connections among the individual parts of your body, and your body as a whole. It is because of *kwăn* that the body communicates with itself. This isn't something we are conscious of; it simply is. For instance, your mind connects to your kidneys, working with them through the kidney *kwăn*. It is a connecting life force. *Kwăn* also maintain function, so it is the *kwăn* of the heart that is the life force that keeps the heart functioning. *Kwăn* also creates

---

47 Possibly other places as well.

connections among the three aspects. *Kwăn* are the commanders, guardians, and protectors of the body, linking the physical body to the mind.

Your *kwăn* is cemented in your body around the fifth month of gestation, and it is the instability or lack of *kwăn* in the fetus that accounts for massage being contraindicated during the first trimester of pregnancy. *Kwăn* are easily scared, injured, or even stolen, and can leave the body during times of trauma, either emotional/energetic/mental or physical. This is called *kwăn hăai* (ขวัญหาย), or "spirit loss."

Sometimes *kwăn hăai* happens to your full *kwăn*, the combination of all the *kwăn*, but it can also happen to a specific smaller *kwăn*. A major trauma such as witnessing the death of your parents or being raped may cause, say, the heart *kwăn* to leave. This will affect your whole being, and the missing *kwăn* must be called back.[48] To hold onto your *kwăn* or to persuade it to return, it is necessary to feel safe and peaceful.

When a person has *kwăn hăai*, those who care about him or her should bring comforting foods, sing soothing songs, and help them to feel loved and cared for. In Thailand, if simple measures do not return the missing *kwăn*, a spirit doctor would be called for to perform a *reeak kwăn* (เรียกขวอัญ), a ceremony that calls the *kwăn* back, but if you do not live where there are spirit doctors readily available, the person with the missing *kwăn* must be nurtured, comforted, warmed, nourished, and swaddled by wrapping them in comforting blankets.

Babies are particularly vulnerable to *kwăn hăai* and so must be kept peaceful and safe at all times. There is a Thai song that parents will sing to their children to call back the *kwăn*. The song goes *kwăn ôie kwăn maa* (ขวัญเอ้ยขวัญมา), "*kwăn*, oh, *kwăn*, come back."

Kwăn is a large reason why it is always important to treat the spiritual when dealing with sickness and imbalance. Say an organ isn't functioning properly, there is a chance that the reason is because the *kwăn* of that organ is missing or injured, so this level of well-being must be addressed. It is common in Thailand to see monks tying white string around people's wrists as a protection for the *kwăn*. This small ceremony is to reinforce the *kwăn* and is called *sòo kwăn* (สู่ขวัญ).

Essence

Essence is said to be a gold-ish colored substance that resides in the body in the heart and is supported by sleep and food, especially food. It gives you your luster and glow and helps support a healthy immune system. Essence is associated with the creation and becoming aspect of Water. It is a life force potential, our vitality and vigor. It is connected to reproduction and the kidneys, but is stored in the heart. When it is depleted we feel weak, depressed, nonvibrant.

Healthy children have a lot of essence, being fully in that becoming, growth stage of life. They have a vibrancy and a glow about them. Women feel a surge of essence when they are ovulating; they lose essence when they menstruate, as the life force creation potential is shed both physically and energetically. This is why menstruation can be such a depleting and difficult

---

48 The heart *kwăn* is frequently a cause of malady. A person with a missing or injured heart *kwăn* may seem disconnected from their body, suffer from depression, and be awkward within themselves.

time. Men lose essence when they ejaculate, sometimes becoming nearly narcoleptic from the depletion of life force potential that has built up within them.

Thai medicine advises men to eat essence-nourishing foods after ejaculation, such as almonds, dates, and honey; women are advised to nourish themselves with blood tonics when they menstruate. We begin to lose essence from the age when we begin to menstruate and ejaculate. Essence is maintained by eating healthily, keeping your kidneys warm, and avoiding depleting activities, such as smoking, drinking, drugs, and overwork. Engaging in healthy and life-affirming activities and getting enough sleep strongly support essence.

Essence is your juicy, vibrant, glowing vitality. It is connected to everything, but especially to the kidneys, the heart, the endocrine system[49] and the immune system. "Endocrine system" and "pituitary gland" are words taken from biomedicine, but they work for our explanatory purpose here. Certain diseases especially deplete essence, such as fevers, which burn up essence.

Release Points
Gòt jùt | กดจุด

Release points are concentrated places that mostly affect the levels of the tissue and sen that can be manipulated to release the surrounding area of tension and blockages. Bodywork systems all over the world have discovered the existence of these points, giving them a variety of names, but they are essentially the same in all cultures. The Thai release point system is spot-specific, however; since many of the release points are on *sên* lines, it makes sense that referral such as "trigger point" work can happen. This is due to the fact that if you remove blockage from one point on a *sên* line the Wind will be freed, thereby potentially affecting other parts of the body.

Wind Gates
Bprà-dtoo lom | ประตูลม

Wind Gate points (*Bprà-dtoo lom*) occur where there is a natural bend in the body (joints). These natural junctions where the path bends also become places where Wind is obstructed and energy and toxins become congested. This can cause a localized problem or a deficiency farther along. Wind Gates are places where we can affect this flow through a gentle resetting of the energy or through more physically intensive work. They are generally found where we can feel the pulse at a joint.

People often associate Wind Gates with arterial pulses, but it is important to remember that what is being addressed here is the Wind, the full flow of movement not just the arteries. The Wind flows through the veins, ligaments, tendons, and nerves as well as the arteries; however, these structures are more difficult to palpate and work directly without engaging the arterial pulse. When we engage the pulse, we are also touching the surrounding *sên*, such as tendons and nerves.

---

49 All of the endocrine system, but especially the pituitary gland, relates to hormones that affect our sense of happiness.

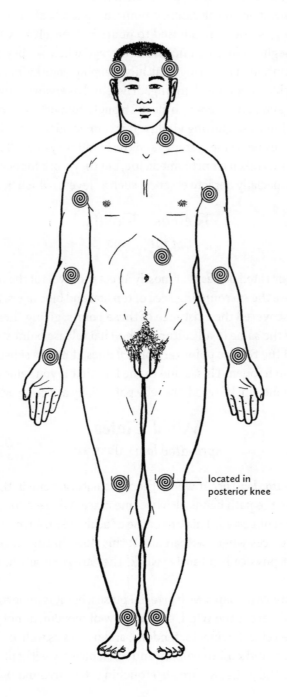

located in
posterior knee

Location of Major Wind Gates

Heart Mind
Jìt jai | จิตใจ

Jìt jai is a combined understanding of the heart and mind, with the two words essentially combining to mean heart, spirit, thoughts, and mind. This connection of mind and heart exists because Thai medicine views thoughts, emotions, consciousness, and spirit as all having an association with the heart, and the heart is the seat of the mind. You can see this heart/mind unity in the Thai language in many common sayings. For example, to "understand" is *kâo jai* (เข้าใจ), meaning "enter heart." Therapies that treat one, treat the other, and imbalances in one are imbalances in the other.

In most forms of traditional medicine thought, feeling, spirit, and such are associated with the heart; yet, of course, we can see how the mind is a participant in these things. In Buddhism, which is the foundation of Traditional Thai Medicine, unharmonious thoughts and emotions are considered one of the causations of disease and imbalance. *Jìt Jai,* then, is often thought to be the root source of all illness. The heart mind is generally treated with fragrant herbs.

Food and Waste Products

The moment we take something into our body, such as food and drink, it becomes a part of the body. Because of this, undigested food is considered one of the thirty-two body parts. Likewise, waste products such as feces and urine are a part of our body until they have been eliminated. Each element has its own waste product, and it is important to eliminate waste from each of them daily. Wind must be eliminated through exhalation, Fire through sweating, Water through urination, and Earth through defecation. It should be noted that what we put into our bodies, and how it looks (smells, feels, and so on) coming out is a significant piece of information used in Thai diagnosis.

CHAPTER THREE

Disease and Imbalance

Various States of the Elements

ELEMENTS CAN EXIST on a spectrum of balance and imbalance that ranges from healthy (balanced) to broken and missing (at which point the person is dying) and many stages in between.

Elemental States	
Som-dun (สมดุล) Balance, healthy, normal	This is the state of being healthy and balanced. Healthy for each individual is unique, however, as our core elemental constitutions will express themselves. One healthy person will be more watery, or windy, or fiery than another.
Gam rêrp (กำเริบ) Excited, agitated, amplified, excessive	An excited element is functioning above normal, over-projecting itself, and dominating the other elements to an unhealthy degree.
Yòn (หย่อน) Weakened, depleted, deficient	A weakened element is functioning below normal and will not assert itself enough. There is a lack of vitality to the weakened element.
Pí-gaan (พิการ) Distorted, deranged	The element is disrupted or distorted. In this state, the element is more disturbed than *gam rêrp* or *yòn,* and may show signs of being both agitated and weakened.
Săn ni-bàat (สันนิบาต) Multiple elements disturbed	The term *Săn ni-bàat* generally refers to when multiple elements have become disturbed and the condition has become quite serious. It can also indicate that the Earth element has become affected, which also indicates that the condition is serious and other elements are disturbed.
Dtaèk (แตก) Broken	A broken element is so weakened that it has stopped functioning. It is still in the body holding space, but it is not doing its job. This is a very serious condition, often fatal and requiring major medical care.
Hăai bpai (หายไป) Disappeared, lost, missing	The moment that an element ceases to exist in the body, it is disappeared. At this point, death is in process, as we cannot live without all of the elements.

Elements in Balance
Som-dun | สมดุล

Traditional Thai Medicine, being a niche branch of Buddhist medicine, contains within it the understanding of impermanence, that all things are constantly subject to and prone to change. This is inclusive of the balance of elements within us, or our state of "health." Because all things are constantly changing, health is not defined by an absence of symptoms. It is natural to go in and out of balance throughout our lives. It is the nature of the body to experience illness, age, and eventually death. Buddhist medicine understands that there is no such thing as an indefinite state of health; therefore, a Thai medicine practitioner can approach disease and discomfort with a calm mental state about it. This cognition of change, including the fluctuation of well-being, as being natural and acceptable, is a first step toward what Buddha called "right thought," and is therefore the first step toward a calm mind.

Within this comprehension that we cannot exist in a stasis of health, we do our best to maintain our body, mind, and environment so as to continually redirect ourselves toward optimal balance and function as unhindered by disease as possible. We do our best to maintain balance among the body, mind, and environment, but a part of being healthy is accepting that illness and death are inevitable; they are the nature of a human birth. Attempting to run from this fact only brings further suffering.

With this in mind, let's explore what a general state of healthy looks like in the varying elements.

Wind (Son-Dun)

When Wind element is healthy and balanced, movement throughout the body is not too fast or too slow. Food moves through the digestive tract at the proper speed, blood circulates at a steady even pace, and there is no excess motion, such as tics and twitches. Balanced Wind results in clear, non-chaotic thinking, a quick grasp of new ideas, and clear speech patterns. All neural synapses, muscle contractions and extensions, and other gross movements in the body are unimpeded.

Fire (Son-Dun)

When Fire element is balanced, the body will have the correct amount of stomach acid for strong yet balanced digestion and nutrients will be properly digested. Body temperature will be healthy, and one will not run too hot or too cold. Balanced Fire will age at the correct rate, meaning that tissue and cells will not deteriorate too fast. Skin will have good color and tone, and will be oily enough but not too oily. Healthy Fire will have good drive, motivation, and willpower, clear strong speech, and an ability to focus.

Water (Son-Dun)

When Water element is normal and healthy, the tissue and skin will be well hydrated, the digestive tract will be properly lubricated, and blood volume will be normal. Saliva will be soothing to the mouth, with normal speech and swallowing. Weight will be balanced, and hair will be healthy. A person with normal Water element should have a healthy ability to be compassionate, nurturing, and calm and have strong vitality.

Earth (Son-Dun)

With a healthy Earth element, all twenty parts of the body made of Earth are strong and healthy. This is the bones, the skin, the hair, the structure of the organs—all of the supporting structures of the body. The tissue will be strong yet flexible, with normal movement. The mind will be calm and balanced.

States of Element Imbalance
Tâat sà-mùt-tăan | ธาตุสมุฏฐาน

The current condition of imbalance, as opposed to the core elemental constitution, is called colloquially in Thai, Tâat bpàt jù bpan (ธาตุปัจจุบัน) or, as I will call it here, Tâat sà-mùt-tăan; which translates as "the elemental disease-causing factor," or more precisely, "elemental causative factor." So if Fire is out of balance, one could say "tâat Fai sà-mùt-tăan."

Regardless of core elemental constitution, what is out of balance is what must be treated, and is therefore of greater importance. As stated earlier, knowing a person's core elemental constitution may be beneficial in understanding just how far out of balance they are; however, what we pay attention to, what we treat, is the imbalance, the Tâat sà-mùt-tăan. Another way of looking at this is to say that we treat what is currently presenting. There are many methods of diagnosis, several of which will be discussed here, but the first thing one needs to do is to become familiar with how elements in different states tend to present.

Now let's spend some time looking at the various states of imbalance that an element can exist in. We will look most closely at Gam rêrp (excited) and Yòn (weakened), as these are the states that bodyworkers will likely work with the most. While the terms "excessive," "depleted," and "deficient" are presented in the chart at the beginning of this chapter as alternate wording for Gam rêrp and Yòn, they must be used with care. When speaking of the element as a system in the body, only the quality of the element, not the quantity, changes. Therefore, most of the time, these quantitive terms are a bit misleading. In most cases, it is more accurate to say that an element is "excited" or "weakened" than to imply that there is more or less of it present.

Sometimes though, we actually have too much or not enough of an element as a body part. For instance, when retaining Water, such as in cases of edema, we can say that someone has an excess of Water that needs to be released from the body by getting the sên and organs to process the Water out of the body properly through sweat and urination. This elemental excess is spot-specific and quite literal, but it stems from excited Water. Another example of this would be heatstroke, in which there is an excess of Fire in the head causing systemic illness and headache. When you scrape[50] the head on someone with heatstroke you can tangibly feel the

---

50 Therapy technique involving rubbing with a tool.

excessive heat (Fire) as it exits the body. For Wind, we can see how excess Wind is expelled in the form of belching and passing gas.

Again, this is connected to, but different from, when we talk about the element as a body system. In these cases, the systemic elemental imbalance has led to an accumulation of the element as a waste product that must be eliminated from the body. So to say that someone has agitated Fire might mean that they have excess heat that needs to be released, but it also might mean that they are systemically fiery: temperamental, digesting food overly fast, or overly driven, to name a few possible outcomes. One state may often lead to another, but clarity about when the word "excess" is used is important.

Excited, Agitated, Amplified, Excessive
Gam rêrp | กำเริบ

An excited element is functioning above normal, over-projecting itself, and dominating the other elements to an unhealthy degree. In most cases, if you think about the qualities, experience, and function of the element, as well as normal characteristics of an element as it manifests in a person's core elemental constitution, this will give you a clue about what it will look like in an overexcited state. All of the normal attributes will be amplified to an unhealthy degree.

Wind (Gam Rêrp)

All conditions involving too much movement, whether it is the movement of a nervous tic, or the movement of thoughts swirling through a mind that will not calm, are attributed to excited Wind element. Some examples would be twitches, spasms, restless leg syndrome, and movement-affected diseases such as Parkinson's disease and multiple sclerosis. Tourette's, whether it manifests in twitches or spontaneous vocalizations, is an excited Wind disorder, as the vocalizations are a movement of sound.

In the digestive system too much Wind can create diarrhea, overly fast movement of food through the digestive tract, causing a lack of absorption of nutrients and hence, malnourishment. Accumulation of Wind in the digestive tract can also be seen in bloating and excessive gas or belching.

Agitated mental Wind causes anxiety and insomnia, with thoughts that will not be still; in more extreme cases, agitated mental Wind will result in mental health disorders such as schizophrenia and psychosis, and the Asperger's end of the autism/Asperger's spectrum. Obsessive compulsive disorders tend to stem from the efforts of a chaotic Windy mind attempting to create order.

In the circulatory system excited Wind will manifest in a fast pulse or heart rate, and in the pulmonary system we may see hyperventilation. Other signals of excessive Wind include fast and chaotic speech patterns, easy overwhelm and overstimulation, an inability to focus, very dry skin, an inability to stay warm, and bluish-gray coloring.[51]

---

51 This is a pale grayish, or bluish, or sometimes blackish color. It is not precise.

Fire *(Gam Rêrp)*

Fire in agitation or excess generally shows itself boldly, with red coloration, hot temperatures, and strong emotions. Fevers, including toxic fevers such as malaria, dengue, and yellow fever, are all symptoms of excessive Fire element. All outward displays of redness, such as rashes, acne, and flushing are also symptomatic of excessive Fire element. Overly strong emotions of anger, frustration, excitement, and passion are attributed to Fire element, as is excessive drive, as seen with workaholics and those who will stop at nothing to achieve their goals. Excessive digestive Fire will cause food to break down too quickly, preventing nutrient absorption, and it can excite digestive Wind, causing diarrhea. The Fire of aging and decay, when excessive, will cause tissue deterioration, rapid cellular decay, and shortened life expectancy. People with agitated Fire generally have a low tolerance for heat and may be prone to heat-based funguses.

Water *(Gam Rêrp)*

Health problems when Water is excited usually arise from mucous in the body, and a primary sign of agitated Water is excessive mucous. This frequently manifests in the head and throat, chest and lungs, or in the lower abdomen. Water out of balance is susceptible to colds, and it can take a long time to get rid of them. This is because Water element is a thick, heavy element. It takes longer to process out toxins and pathogens, and is associated with a generally slower metabolism. Along these lines, when Water is too thick it becomes stagnant and collects toxins. Sexual dysfunctions and kidney or urinary infections are often at least in part due to Water imbalance. Excessive Water also shows up in damp overly hydrated skin and tissue, and Water retention such as edema. When Water is agitated it often leads to weight gain, lethargy, and slowness of both physical and mental processes. Extreme emotions of depression, sadness, nostalgia, and melancholy are signs of agitated Water, and in extreme cases, mental Water imbalance can manifest as Down's syndrome or the autism end of the autism/Asperger's spectrum.

Earth *(Gam Rêrp)*

Being the heaviest/densest and least malleable element, Earth is the last element that is affected by imbalance. By the time the Earth element is affected, we are usually talking about a fully manifested disease and not just a small imbalance. People with a lot of Earth element are not often ill, but once Earth is affected it can be extremely difficult to remedy, as it is likely to manifest as cancers, tumors, and other excesses in matter, although there are excesses of matter that are not so serious, such as benign moles and nonharmful bone spurs. The Earth element can also be directly impacted by things such as weapons and accidents. In this case, there is no disease progression through the other elements, as something like a car accident can instantly damage the Earth parts of the body, such as bones, tissue, and organs. Agitated Earth element in someone can cause stagnation, obesity, lethargy, stubbornness, and a failure to grow and change.

Weakened, Depleted, Deficient
Yòn | หย่อน

A weakened element is functioning below normal and will not assert itself enough. There is a lack of vitality to the weakened element. Again if we think about the qualities, experience, and function of the element, we can guess how a person might be affected when the element is weakened, as these qualities will be lacking or insufficient.

Wind *(Yòn)*

Weakened Wind is implicated anytime there is a lack of healthy mobility. This includes tissue rigidity, paralysis, slow mental processes, neural impediment, and conditions such as amyotrophic lateral sclerosis (ALS). Deficient Wind element can cause food to move too slowly through the digestive tract. This allows the food to ferment and become toxic, which in turn can lead to a variety of other problems, from malnourishment to inflammation and pain. Weakened Wind can also cause low blood pressure, poor circulation, and resulting fatigue and fainting. With depleted Wind, one might feel mentally slow and uncreative.

Fire *(Yòn)*

Weakened Fire can cause low body temperature, pale skin, and lack of vitality. It also often leads to poor digestion due to low digestive fire/insufficient stomach acid. When food cannot be properly broken down, we cannot absorb the nutrients, which leads to malnourishment, and the food ferments inside of us, leading to excess Wind in the digestive tract and toxins that travel throughout the body causing inflammation, often in the joints. Unhealthy Fire can also result in low red blood cell count. When the Fire of aging and decay is weakened, there is a lower rate of tissue deterioration, resulting in conditions such as thick skin and tongue. Weak Fire often causes a lack of motivation, self-preservation, courage, and willpower, and those without healthy Fire element are likely to be physically weak.

Water *(Yòn)*

With weakened Water element there may not be enough mucous in the digestive system. This can lead to hard feces, scraping the colon, and painful defecation. Weakened Water can also cause poor blood volume, in which case the blood vessels will feel hard and wirelike, and one may suffer from headaches. Deficient Water can cause the mouth to have insufficient saliva, resulting in dryness, discomfort, foul breath, thirst, dry throat, and possibly blood in the mouth. Skin and tissue will be dry in cases of depleted Water, and the joints will lack lubrication. Reproductive issues, such as infertility and sexual problems, are frequently found with weakened Water element. People with insufficient Water are likely to be ungrounded, anxious, and show signs of heightened Fire element. They may also experience trouble staying focused or maintaining a chain of thought.

Earth *(Yón)*

Deficient Earth element is associated with any weakening in the Earth parts of the body. This may be seen in tissue degeneration, osteoporosis, thin skin, and structural instability and frailty. Conditions such as ulcers, damage to the structure of the liver or other organs, weak brittle nails, soft teeth, and easily torn tendons and ligaments are all examples of weak Earth. Insufficient Earth element will also cause a person to be ungrounded and prone to excessive emotions.

As you can see, with *gam rêrp* and *yón*, oftentimes one element being excited will look like another element that is weakened, and a weakened element may look like another element that is excited. It can take time to be able to see what is actually going on, and if both, what is the root problem.

Distorted, Deranged
Pi-gaan | พิการ

Elements in a state of *pi-gaan* are a step beyond a basic imbalance and have begun to display erratic behavior. They may be in a state of fluctuation, oscillating between *gam-rêrp* and *yón*, or exist in both states at once. An example of this is with people with distorted Wind imbalance who have excessive ascending wind (seen in mental windiness, insomnia, restlessness, and so on), yet have deficient descending wind, causing constipation. Because Wind is so easily pulled out of balance, it is the element that more frequently ends up in a state of derangement, so it is very common to find Wind-imbalanced people displaying the above combination.

Another example of elements in derangement would be heart arrhythmia, where the heart beats erratically. Fire element in distortion might be seen in someone who has fever and chills, fluctuating quickly between excessive and deficient Fire. *Pi-gaan* does not have to be a vacillation between strong or weak elemental behavior. It is also used simply to mean that the element is more strongly out of balance than with normal excitement or weakness.

Multiple Elements Disturbed
Săn ni-bàat | สันนิบาต

The next stage of imbalance is *săn-ná-bàat*, in which Water, Fire, and Wind are all disturbed. An example of this would be flu with fever, chills, and vomiting. In this case, Fire and Wind are deranged and Water is deficient. *Săn-ná-bàat* may also present when you see someone who has multiple diseases manifesting at once.

Broken
Dtaèk | แตก

Once an element is broken, in many cases this is very serious and occurs just before death. Broken Wind element can present as circulatory failure, unconsciousness, paralysis, or a failure to breathe. Broken Fire element can be seen in the cessation of bile production. Broken Water element is seen in the dying process, when people no longer produce saliva. And broken Earth element can be seen in structural damage to organs. Broken Earth that is less serious would could be broken bones and muscular atrophy.

Disappeared, Missing
Hăai bpai | หายไป

Hăai bpai comes with death. We must have all of our elements to live, so when one is gone, they all go. For instance, if we have no Fire, as with extreme hypothermia, or no breath of respiration, we cannot live. When we die, our elements return to the elements of the world. The Earth of us decomposes into dirt. The Water (fluids) in us join the waters of the world. Our last breath, the Wind, dissipates into the winds of the world, and the Fire, the last heat of our being, is transferred through conduction from being the heat of our body to the warmth in the world.

Three Stages of Elemental Imbalance

Wíp-bpà-rìt | วิปริต

When an element is disturbed, it is said to be Wíp-bpà-rìt. There are three stages of Wíp-bpà-rìt: beginning, progressing, and broken.

Châat | ชาติ

STAGE ONE: In this stage the imbalance is just starting out, beginning, or accumulating. In the beginning your body will crave that which will bring it into balance.

Jàláná | จะละนะ

STAGE TWO: In this stage, the imbalance is progressing, moving along, continuing. If you do not listen to your body in Stage One, eventually the imbalance takes over and you begin to crave that which feeds it. You can see this in people with excited Fire who crave spicy foods, or people with excited Wind who "feel better" when they do things like fasting, even though realistically fasting will only make them more windy.

Pinná | ภินนะ

STAGE THREE: In this stage the element that is out of balance is completely distorted or broken. The literal translation of pinná is "perverted" or "distorted." In this third stage of imbalance the person is affected by the imbalance, truly feeling the ill effects.

Element Imbalance Causation

There are many possible causes of disease or imbalance, and Thai medicine has various approaches to interpreting causes of suffering, with many different lists and facets breaking down variants of imbalance etiologies.

In the following section, we will look at some of the most useful causative paradigms of imbalance including:

- The Three Causes of Imbalance
- The Four Causes of Imbalance
- External and Internal Causes of Imbalance
- The Three Defilements
- Condensation Through the Layers of the Physical Body
- Other Factors in Disease Origination

Three Causes of Imbalance

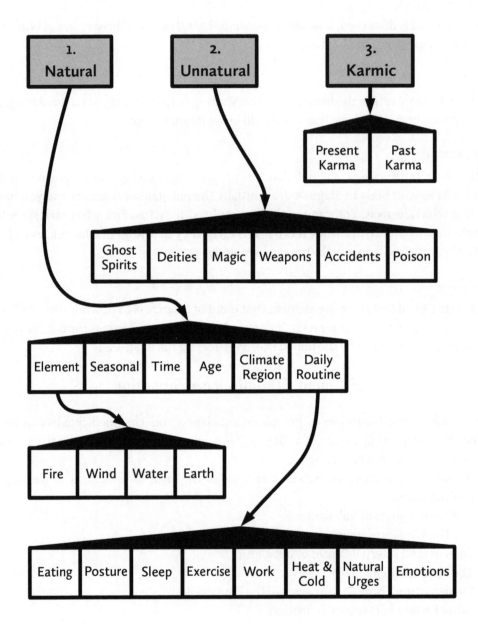

The Three Causes of Imbalance are natural causes of imbalance, unnatural causes of imbalance, and karmic causes of imbalance. I'm beginning with the Three Causes of Imbalance, because this is the most extensive imbalance causation list, and provides a very thorough picture of diagnosis. As I now break down the Three Causes of Imbalance, I highly recommend that you glance at the flow chart above from time to time in order to stay in touch with where we are.

Three sounds like a small number, I know, but this is a list with sublists nested within. Keep in mind that we are going to be spending some time on this one list, before moving on to the other paradigms of imbalance etiology. Don't let the sublists within this list confuse you into thinking we are already on a new causation list entirely.

Natural Causes of Imbalance

The first four natural causes of imbalance are of particular importance in diagnosing disorders. It is said in the traditional medicine text *Phrakhamphii Samutthahn Winitchai* that all disease arises from these four factors:

1. Elemental Causative Factor
Tâat-sù mú-tăan | ธาตุสมุฏฐาน

The elemental causative factor represents the element that is out of balance in the elemental systems within us, or an imbalance between the internal and external elements. The four elemental causative factors are Fire Causative Factor, Wind Causative Factor, Water Causative Factor, and Earth Causative Factor.

As we move into this section, to stay true to traditional Thai teachings, we'll use the words *bpìt-dtà*, *Wâata*, and *Săym-hà*, which stem from the Pali words *pitta*, *vāta*, and *semha*. These words are also found in Ayurvedic medicine; however, it should be noted that the words predate both medical systems and they did not evolve to have exactly the same meaning in Ayurvedic medicine as they came to have in Thai medicine. Let's look more closely at the elemental causative factors.

a. **FIRE CAUSATIVE FACTOR** (*Sà-mùt-tăan dtay-choh-tâat pí-gàt* | สมุฏฐานเตโชธาตุพิกัต)
Fire causative factor is when an imbalance of the Fire element causes suffering. The four forms of Fire—Fire that warms the body, Fire of aging and decay, Fire of emotion and fever, and Fire of digestion are simply components of the body. While they can become weak or agitated, they are not the cause of imbalance themselves. When we talk about Fire as a causative factor, a disease-causing agent, we look at three specific aspects of Fire. These are:

i. **Pát-tá-bpìt-dtà** (พัทธะปิตตะ): *Pát-tá* means "bound" or "contained." *Bpìt-dtà* can mean "bile" or it can be an expression of Fire. *Pát-tá-bpìt-dtà* is *bpìt-dtà* contained or in its seat, such as bile in the digestive tract or the gallbladder, or simply contained as a Fire system in the body.

ii. **A-pát-tá-bpìt-dtà** (อพัทธะปิตตะ): *A-pát-tá* means "unbound," so *A-pát-tá-bpìt-dtà* is unbound *bpìt-dtà*. This is Fire existing where it is not supposed to be, such as with acid reflux or bile in the large intestine. It can also be more systemic—in the blood or the skin, for example.

iii. **Gam-dao** (กาเดา): *Gam-dao* means "body heat" (it also can mean "bloody nose" but not in this application). So here we are talking about things like fever and anger. *Gam-dao* is the most important of the disease-causing aspects of Fire, as maintaining proper body temperature is vitally important.

b. **WIND CAUSATIVE FACTOR** (*Sà-mùt-tăan waa-yoh-tâat pí-gàt* | สมุฏฐานวาโยธาตุพิกัต)
This is when Wind imbalance brings about suffering. Like the four Fires, the six Winds (ascending, descending, and so on) are simply component parts of our being and are not problematic unto themselves. The aspects where Wind carries more potential to become disease-causing agents are the heart Wind, the knife-like Wind, and the central channel Wind.

i. **Heart Wind** (*Hà-tai Wâata* | หทัยวาต): This Wind is the system that is formed from the combination of the Wind that circulates throughout the body and the Wind of respiration. It is located in the heart, made of gross and subtle winds, and spreads emotions, feelings, thoughts, and circulation throughout the body.

ii. **Knifelike Wind** (*Sat-ta-haka Wâata* | สัตถะกะวาต): This is the Wind in the digestive system and the Wind that causes pain. *Sat-ta-haka* can also be translated as "piercing." A common experience of *Sat-ta-haka Wâata* disease would be the sharp pains of too much gas in the digestive tract. While inflammation comes from Fire, and swelling comes from Water, all pain is attributed to Wind.

iii. **Central Channel Wind** (*Sù má naa Wâata* | สุมะนาวาต): This is the Wind in the central part of the body. It is made of the descending and ascending winds, resides in the spinal cord, inferior and superior vena cavas, and the ascending and descending aortas. This Wind is said to be the most important, in that it maintains the whole body and is supported by the other Winds.

c. **WATER CAUSATIVE FACTOR** (*Sà-mùt-tăan aa-bpoh pí-gàt* | สมุฏฐานอาโปพิกัต)
Water Causative Factor is when an imbalance of the Water element causes suffering. As with Fire and Wind, the twelve Water components of the body (bile, mucous, pus, and so on) are not problematic unto themselves. The potential disease-causing aspects of Water are the mucous of the neck and head, mucous of the chest and abdomen, and mucous of the lower abdomen.

i. **Mucous in the Neck and Head** (*Sŏr Săym-hà* | ศอเสมหะ): *Sŏr Săym-hà* refers to the mucous in the neck and head, although some texts say between the diaphragm and the head.

ii. **Mucous in the Chest and Abdomen** (*U-rá Săym-hà* | อุระเสมหะ): *U-rá Săym-hà* is mucous related to the chest and the abdomen, but primarily the chest.

iii. **Mucous in the Bowels** (*Kuut Săym-hà* คูธเสมหะ): *Kuut Săym-hà* is mucous related to the lower abdomen, especially in the bowels.

d. **EARTH CAUSATIVE FACTOR** (*Sà-mùt-tăan bpà-tà-wĕe tâat pí-gàt* | สมุฏฐานปถวีธาตุพิกัต)
Earth Causative Factor is when an imbalance in the Earth element is causing suffering. The twenty parts of Earth as component parts in the body can become affected, but they are not

the cause. The disease-causing aspects of Earth element are the organs, new food in the body, and old food/fecal matter.

i. **Heart** (*Hà-tai wát-tù* หทัยวัตถุ): *Hà-tai* means "heart," and *wát-tù* means "components, things, or pieces." In this context, what is meant is the physical heart as well as the other organs.

ii. **New Food** (*Ù-tá-rí-yá* | อุทริยะ): *Ù-tá-rí-yá* is "new food in the stomach, the bolus." Some say this word means "the stomach." The *Ù-tá-rí-yá*, the food you take into your body, has a huge effect on the whole body. It goes on to become the body, so it's very important what you eat. Also, the organ of the stomach itself must have structural integrity.

iii. **Old Food** (*Gà-rì-sà* | กรีส) *Gà-rì-sà* is "old food in the body, or fecal matter." The health of the bowels and your excrement is probably the key diagnosis of the body and Earth. For this reason, *Gà-rì-sà* is the most important of these three disease-causing agents.

2. Seasonal Causative Factor

A-dtù-sù mú-dtà-tăan | อุตุสมุฏฐาน

Seasonal Causative Factor refers to the natural amplification of certain elements based on the season. It is natural for Fire to be stronger during hot seasons, Wind to be stronger during rainy seasons,[52] and Water to be stronger during cold seasons. These natural fluctuations, however, easily go too far, leading to imbalance.

3. Time Causative Factor

gaan-sù mú-dtà-tăan | กาลสมุฏฐาน

Time Causative Factor refers to both the time of day and astrological times, hence astrology is included in the Time Causative Factor. The Time Causative Factor is due to how different elements are stronger at different times of day, with Wind element being dominant in the early morning, Water element being dominant in the late morning, and Fire element being dominant at midday. The pattern then repeats itself in the second half of the day, with Wind being dominant in early afternoon, Water being dominant in late afternoon, and Fire being dominant in the middle of the night.

4. Age Causative Factor

aa-yú-sù mú-dtà-tăan | อายุสมุฏฐาน

The Age Causative Factor reflects how different elements rule different times of life. Water is naturally stronger in childhood, Fire is naturally stronger from the teens until the early thirties, and Wind is naturally stronger in later life. While these changes are natural, they can cause imbalance. The element that dominates a certain age period in life is called the *tâat jâo reuan* (ธาตเจ้าเรือน), which translates to "the lord, or master, of the house."

---

52 Most people assume that Water is stronger during rainy seasons; however, rain is associated with strong winds, and even the movement of rain connects to Wind. Cold, on the other hand, is a quality of Water, hence cold seasons are when Water is strong.

This term has been used in more recent times to refer to the core elemental constitution (see diagnosis chapter), but traditionally only applies to the age causative factor.

Age & Elements		Season & Elements		Time & Elements	
Birth to 8 yrs	Water	**Hot Season**	Fire	2 a.m.-6 a.m.	Wind
8 yrs. to 16 yrs	Water waning, Fire waxing	**Rainy Season** (in some countries, spring and fall)	Water	6 a.m. - 10 a.m.	Water
16 yrs. to 32 yrs	Fire			10 a.m. - 2 p.m.	Fire
32 yrs to 64 yrs	Fire waning, Wind waxing	**Cold Season**	Wind	2 p.m. - 6 p.m.	Wind
64 yrs and up	Wind			6 p.m. - 10 p.m.	Water
				10 p.m. - 2 a.m.	Fire

5. Region/Climate

bprà-tâyt-sù mú-dtà-tăan | ประเทศสมุฏฐาน

Hot dry climates increase Wind and Fire. Hot, wet climates increase Water or Fire. Cold, wet climates increase Water and/or Wind. And cold climates increase Water.

6. Daily Routine (Eight Daily Habits)

This is the most common cause of imbalance. Chapter nine elaborates on healthy daily habits for each elemental make up. Daily routine consists of eight daily habits:

a. *Eating Habits:* Too much food, too little food, eating at the wrong time, eating foods that are incorrect for your elemental makeup, and eating bad quality food all lead to imbalance.

b. *Posture:* Staying in one position for too long, not alternating between postures, and habitually holding the body in poor posture all lead to imbalance.

c. *Sleep Habits:* Too much sleep, too little sleep, poor quality sleep, and sleeping at the wrong times are common causes of imbalance.

d. *Exercise:* Exercising too hard, at the wrong time of day, or doing exercises that are not appropriate for your elemental makeup cause imbalance.

e. *Work:* Working harder than the body and/or mind can handle causes elemental imbalance, as does working jobs that are not enjoyable over the long term.

f. *Extremes of Temperature:* Being in places that are very hot or very cold, or going from one temperature extreme to another, such as the hot desert outside to the cold air-conditioned office, is a common cause of illness.

g. **Suppression of Natural Urges:** Suppressing bodily actions such as urination, defecation, sneezing, passing gas, yawning, and burping leads to elemental imbalance.

h. **Emotions:** Excessive strong emotions, including excessive sadness, depression, anger, sorrow, or even joy will eventually lead to imbalance.

Unnatural Causes of Imbalance

Unnatural causes of imbalance is the second of the Three Causes of Imbalance. Imbalances stemming from unnatural causes include:

- **Ghosts and Spirits** - Ghosts and spirits can cause imbalance through possessions, or simply through their presence, which frequently affects Wind. Having ghosts around is much like having a draft.
- **Deities** - Deities can inflict disease. This generally happens when someone creates a connection to a deity and then breaks it, especially if the connection came with vows.
- **Magic** - Hexes and other magical interventions can cause imbalance. In Thailand, there is strong belief that many troubles are caused by hexes, but my teacher says that this is less common than people think.
- **Weapons** - Imbalance is generally directly related to Earth element when the body is injured by weapons, with other elements being affected secondarily.
- **Accidents** - Imbalance is generally directly related to Earth element when the body is injured through accidents, with other elements being affected secondarily
- **Poison** - Poisons can cause imbalance to varying elements, depending on the poison.

Karmic Causes of Imbalance

Karmic causes are the third of the Three Causes of Imbalance. Karma is often found to be the cause of very stubborn disorders that do not respond to any treatment.

- **Past Karma** - This is not a punishment; it is simply the natural laws of cause and effect in motion.
- **Present Karma** - This is also not punishment, but the current effects of our actions and reactions.

This concludes the section on the Three Causes of Imbalance. Please note that the following lists are separate approaches to imbalance causation. There is some overlap between the lists, but different lists are provided as there is not one list that presents every possible pathology etiology.

Four Causes of Imbalance

The Four Causes of Imbalance is a somewhat simpler list of disease causation, with much over-lap from the Three Causes of Imbalance list.

1. Imbalances from within the body

When all is well, the elements act as harmonious systems within us. However, when they go out of balance we can have systemic internal elemental imbalance. This is similar to the elemental Causative Factor presented and elaborated on in the Three Causes of Imbalance.

2. External factors, such as climate and pathogens

This is the influence of weather, geography, exposure to germs and any other pathogens from the external world.

3. Unseen forces, such as black magic, ghosts, deities, and spirits

This includes possessions, hexes, influences from deities and other metaphysical forces.

4. Astrological Influences, Age, and Time

As in the Three Causes of Imbalance, we see here that planetary alignment, time of day, and time of life all have influence upon our elemental makeup.

External and Internal Causes of Imbalance

Much of this list is reflected in the lists above; however, this can be a helpful list for under-standing imbalance origination.

- *Imbalances Resulting From Problems with Internal Balance*
  Internal balance refers to the balance of the elements and systems of the body. When all is balanced internally, there should be no physical manifestations of imbalance. Many minor internal imbalances, such as imbalances with Wind, can be brought into equilibrium with physical therapies.
- *Imbalance Resulting From External Substance Being Taken Into the Body*
  The most common example of the intake of substances reacting with the internal body is food. When we eat foods that are not correct for us, indigestion and gas can result. External therapies such as bodywork can remedy this. If incorrect eating is habitual it will result in bigger problems, ranging from joint inflammation to structural damage to the body such as ulcers. In addition to food, unclean air taken in through respiration, excessive jarring or unpleasant sounds taken in through the ears, and disturbing visions can all affect our elemental balance.
- *Imbalances Resulting From External Substance Affecting The Outer Body*
  External substances affecting the outer body refers to a pathway of imbalance in which a pathogen such as a cool wind, intense sun, or germs enter the body through the skin, then progress through the layers of the physical body. This can be a particularly important imbalance path for bodyworkers to be aware of and work with.

The Three Defilements

The three defilements are seen as the root, or umbrella cause, of all imbalance. They reflect the Buddhist nature of Thai medicine and will be elaborated on in Chapter Seven. For the first two, more than one word is used to describe the defilement due to there not being a direct single word translation.

1. *Greed/Lust:* Greed and lust tend to be associated with Wind imbalances.
2. *Hatred/Aversion:* Hatred and aversion tend to be associated with Fire imbalances.
3. *Delusion:* Delusion tends to be associated with Water imbalances.

The three defilements are ultimately caused by not knowing—not knowing truth, not knowing or understanding the reality of the way things are. This is said to keep us in the life cycle and leads to disease and suffering.

Condensation Through the Layers of the Physical Body

Here we see a merging of the five layers of the physical body—skin, tissue, sên, bone, and organs—and the concept of how elements condense and dissipate.

1. Skin

The skin is an organ of both elimination and absorption. This means that it acts like a door through which pathogens can both enter the body and be released from the body. In a healthy body the skin acts as a layer of defense, allowing pathogens and waste (sweat) out of the body but acting as a barrier to pathogens getting in. However, when we are weakened, the skin cannot do its job properly. When a pathogen such as heat or cold (anyone who has had heatstroke from the sun or bound muscles from the cold can understand how heat and cold are pathogens) enters through the skin, it quickly goes to the next layer, the tissue.

2. Tissue

When, for example, a chill wind has entered through the skin layer, it can quickly permeate to the layer of muscle and fascia, creating binding and spasm in the tissue, as well as aching, pain, and adhesions. These are often easily taken care of through bodywork therapies such as massage, scraping, and cupping; however, if this is allowed to persist it will progress to the *sên*.

3. Sên

Let's continue with the example of the chill wind. Once it has entered the tissue layer, the constriction of the muscle and fascia will lead to blockages of the *sên* and therefore blockage of the Wind element in the body. This means that blood and lymph are not flowing properly; movement in the muscles, tendons, and ligaments is impeded; and possibly nerves are impinged. All of this blockage in the *sên* is going to lead to stagnation and a buildup of toxins. Any movement that continues in the *sên* is going to spread these toxins throughout the body to the bone.

4. Bone

In the example we are following, the layer of the bone is primarily affected in the joints, where the toxins become stuck due to the natural curve in the path. This is a very common area to experience pain, stuck Wind, and inflammation. To bring in the example of heatstroke, in this case we very quickly experience achy joints and nausea, as the pathogens progress fast to the layer of the organs.

5. Organs

The organs are the last layer of the body affected in this particular imbalance path (whereas with intake of substances such as food, smoke, and alcohol, they can be first), and oftentimes they are not reached at all. If they are reached, the hollow organs (those connecting directly to the external such as the stomach and lungs) are affected first, with the solid (land-locked) organs next.

Understanding how pathogens condense down through the layers of the physical body, we can see how physical therapies can be used to free the tissue and *sên* of blockages with massage, beating, cupping, herbal therapies, and so on; loosen and lubricate the joints through range of motion, traction, and bone setting; and draw pathogens such as heat and toxins out through the skin with therapies such as cupping, scraping, and application of drawing liniments. Bodyworkers essentially go through the first few body layers and break up the congestion, dissipating what was condensed. Some of this travels through the *sên* into the core, to be processed by the organs, and some is brought to the surface, where the skin can do its job as an organ of elimination.

Other Factors in Disease Origination

Wastes

Each element creates and must eliminate waste every day. Wind waste is eliminated through exhaled breath. Fire waste is eliminated through perspiration. Water waste is eliminated through urination. And Earth waste is eliminated through defecation. If the elemental wastes are not eliminated, this can be a source of imbalance.

Losing Essence

We use the words "depletion" or "depleted" a lot, but we don't often take the time to unpack them. This is because really, we all know what they mean. We understand pretty intrinsically what a depleted person is—weak, tired, unhealthy, low energy, often low emotionally. We can get more specific, talking about someone being depleted in a certain element, vitamin, sleep, or sunlight—all the things we need to survive well. But this is usually a beginning point.

Depletion in one thing usually snowballs into a general depletion. Lack of sleep may affect digestion, and now you have lack of food nourishment, which translates to a lack of vitamins, minerals, fats, and so on. What we are really talking about, ultimately, is essence being depleted, because depletion of any single life-sustaining nutrient (counting sleep, exercise, sunlight, and all the things we need as "nutrients" here) is going to deplete our essence. There are natural ways as well as unnatural ways in which we lose essence.

Some natural ways that we lose essence
- Ejaculation
- Menstruation
- Childbirth
- Growing old

Some unnatural ways that we lose essence
- Lack of nutrition (either through eating unhealthy food, or from having problems in your digestive system that prevent proper food breakdown and absorption)
- Lack of sleep
- Working too hard
- Drug use
- Smoking
- Too much or too little exercise
- Too much strong emotion
- Engaging in life activities that are not fulfilling
- Stress

In the natural list, the first three can be mitigated. With ejaculation, of course, men can control how often it occurs in order to find balance between healthy and depleting forms.[53] Menstruation cannot be controlled without the use of medicines, but we can do things to feed essence around this time. Depletion from childbirth can be mitigated by women doing restorative therapies. There is, of course, nothing to be done about growing old; it is simply the natural way of life. But you can take longevity tonics (beginning before you are old) and nourish your being with healthy daily habits and nutrients.

Elements (Again!)

The first thing to do when you think about a disease causation and the elements, is to think about the experience, function, then the qualities of the elements. For example, if you know that Wind is a very light element, you can see how behaviors that make you lighter, such as fasting, could agitate the Wind element. Likewise, if we think of how Fire is hot, we can see that basking in the sun and eating spicy foods might agitate the Fire element. Of course, you can also use this knowledge to bring about healing, as when someone whose Fire is weakened is encouraged to do these things not to agitate Fire but to nourish it (but we'll get to that later).

Wind

Basically, anything can cause Wind imbalances. This is why our daily routine is so important to manage in order to be in optimal health. Too much sleep, too little sleep, eating at irregular times, not eating when one is hungry, or holding in urges such as burping, sneezing, hunger,

---

53 Different amounts of sexual activity are recommended for different elemental makeups. Sex is always somewhat depleting, but it can also be nourishing, depending on the situation.

thirst, urination, or defecation. Think of the nature of Wind. It's very light and subtle so it can be easily changed or knocked out of balance. My teachers says that someone can cause a Wind imbalance by looking at you wrong, and I suspect that most people who read this sentence will immediately know what he means. All those things that we do daily are potential factors in distorting Wind if they are done in unhealthy ways.

Wind also becomes agitated with travel, life upheaval (moving, divorce, times of great stress), and during times when it is extra windy out. Other causes of Wind imbalance include digestion and the balance of Fire and Water. Digestion affects Wind because mal-digested food ferments inside the body, causing the often painful digestive Wind of flatulence, bloating, and belching. The balance of Fire and Water can also affect Wind. This is because Fire and Water act as the balance for Wind. They can be likened to positive and negative charges—between these two charges, electricity is created. We can liken electricity to Wind, and see that Wind can be created by Fire and Water. Wind can become weakened due to an abundance of Earth or Water weighing the person down, a lack of movement, or exhaustion.

Fire

Some of the factors that can cause Fire to become agitated include overexposure to sun, a diet focused on heating foods such as peppers and other warming spices, diseases that lead to fever, living in hot climates, and holding onto anger and frustration. Fire can also be agitated by a lack of Water element. Fire is weakened by poor diet; lack of exposure to sun; living in cold, dark climates; and agitated Water or Wind elements.[54]

Water

Some causes of Water agitation are poor diet, such as eating too many cold, heavy, and sweet foods; living in a cold and/or wet climate; and sleeping too much.Water can be weakened by dehydration, lethargy, lack of exercise, or agitated Fire or Wind elements.

Earth

Earth element is not easily brought out of balance. It is primarily agitated due to the other elements existing in a state of imbalance for a long time. Earth is weakened due to poor diet, toxins such as steroids that weaken bone and skin, and accidents or warfare that cause trauma to the body.

How Elements Out of Balance Affect One Another

Wind, Fire, or Water can become unbalanced at any time due to multiple factors that will be detailed in chapter three. Earth element, with the exception of sudden trauma to the structural components of the body (such as accidents that cause broken skin, bones, and tissue), is relatively stable and does not go out of balance until some time after all of the other elements have been compromised.

---

54 Agitated Wind can also fan the Fire into excitement. Just as blowing on a flame can extinguish it, with just the right amount of blowing, Wind can be used to increase fire, as seen with the use of bellows on a fireplace.

In most cases, once any one element of Wind, Fire, or Water is unbalanced, it can only stay unbalanced for a certain amount of time before it will affect the health of the other elements. Fire has up to seven days that it can be compromised before it affects the balance of another element, Wind has ten days, and Water has twelve days. When one or two elements are affected, returning to a state of health is not too difficult. However, if remedial measures are not taken, by the end of twenty-nine days (one lunar cycle), in most cases all three of the more malleable elements—Wind, Fire, and Water—will become imbalanced.

The state of being of having three elements affected is called *Săn ni-bàat* (สันนิบาต). When the elements are in *Săn ni-bàat* this is a critical time for medical care. It may be difficult to treat imbalance at this point, but it is still quite possible. *Săn ni-bàat* will eventually lead to Earth element becoming distorted. This point, when all four elements are imbalanced, is called *Maha Săn ni-bàat* (มหาสันนิบาต). With *Maha Săn ni-bàat,* treatment is still possible but it is much harder, as once Earth element becomes affected it usually manifests as a very serious condition such as tumors, organ damage, bone disease, and so on.

Wind, Fire and Water have various possible effects upon one another. Because Fire and Water are opposing forces, they are the only ones that have a predictable relationship, as agitated Fire will always cause weakened Water, and agitated Water will always cause weakened Fire. There is a classic example used with element theory in various traditions to explain how the elements are interdependent. In this example, we look at a pot of soup cooking over a fire. The soup (Water element) is held in the pot (Earth element) heated by the fire below (Fire element), which is coaxed into flames by the wind (Wind element). When all elements are happy and in harmony all is well. But if the fire is too low, the soup will ferment instead of cooking. If the fire is too strong, the soup will boil over and dry out, and if it is very strong, it will crack the pot. If the wind is too weak the fire will die, but if the wind is too strong, it will blow the fire out. If there is too much soup in the pot, it will spill over and extinguish the fire. And so on and so forth.

Diagnosis

When I was living in Thailand, there was a time during which I was having a lot of trouble with dogs. I had been chased by a pack of them, and bitten while in the States. The soi dogs [55] in my neighborhood were extra growly with me, and I had become jittery around all pooches, which made me sad since I've always enjoyed ego around being good with animals. One day I asked a spirit doctor about this and he in turn asked me what year I was born, meaning what zodiac animal am I? "That explains it," he said. "You are a rooster. Of course the dogs chase you!"

In a bodywork practice, most of the time we treat fairly clear conditions, such as bound-up muscle tissue, limited range of motion, or injuries such as sprains and strains. Doing traditional disease diagnosis doesn't always come into play; in fact, in many places, massage therapists are not allowed to use terminology such as "diagnosis" since they are not medical doctors. This book, however, treats bodywork as an integral part of traditional medicine, and traditional

---

55 Soi is the Thai word for small neighborhood streets. "Soi dogs" refers to the abundant strays who wander the streets.

medicine does not separate bodywork from other therapies in the same way that modern Western healing arts do. While you may focus on physical therapies, in Thailand, if you are a healer, then you are expected to know how to diagnose a wide range of pathologies through the traditional medicine lens and also have understanding of all five roots of Thai medicine.

In this section we will look at several diagnostic approaches. Some traditional doctors are extremely proficient at using one technique to diagnose imbalance, such as only using pulse diagnosis or tongue diagnosis to determine the cause of suffering. Most people will employ several approaches, as figuring out what is amiss with someone is much like solving a mystery and the more clues you can gather the better. Even doctors who have a strong affinity for one form of diagnosis are advised to employ as many forms as possible to be certain. Since everyone has all the elements within them, you will see each element asserting itself. It is the job of the traditional doctor to look for a preponderance of evidence to determine which element (or elements) is misbehaving.

Five Sense Diagnosis

Bpan-jà in-see | ปัญจอินทรีย์)

We will begin with Five Sense Diagnosis because this gives us the big picture. Traditionally, five sense diagnosis utilized our senses of hearing, sight, touch, smell, and taste to understand what is going on with a patient; however, in modern times, the sense of taste is not often employed. Five sense diagnosis should always be employed even if other forms of diagnosis are utilized.

Hearing

We use hearing for two purposes: listening to the manner of speech and listening to garner information.

TO LISTEN TO THE MANNER OF SPEECH – This is about paying attention to how a person talks to you, as you look for clues as to what element is dominating or is perhaps weak. Wind (Constitution or Excited) tends to speak in a fast and unfocused manner, changing subjects quickly, or using a lot of words and side tracks to get to the point. Wind can be cautious, in the manner of those who are easily overstimulated and therefore are careful not to overwhelm others. When Wind is weak, speech will be slow and thick.

- FIRE (Constitution or Excited) speaks with focus and clarity, sometimes with aggression or passion, and tends to be loud. Fire is generally on point, direct, and can be insensitive. When Fire is weak, speech can be hesitant, unfocused, slow, and overly quiet.
- WATER tends to speak slowly and thoughtfully. When Water is weak, speech can be too direct, reckless, or unfocused.
- EARTH speaks with a deep, resonant voice that is thoughtful, slow, and secure. Weak Earth may speak quickly and with an ungrounded quality. We see here, as we will everywhere, that one element weakened, resembles another element excited. It can be confusing to ascertain which element needs attention, but with time and practice it will become more clear.

TO LISTEN FOR INFORMATION - This occurs during the intake at the beginning of a treatment session, when the patient tells us what is wrong and answers all of our questions about the situation. It is during this time that we are able to employ our Listening to the Manner of Speech skills as well. I always begin by simply asking the person what they want to tell me about their body and being. I will then ask possibly a handful of questions, possibly a laundry list. It depends on how clear or unclear the situation is.

You can use the Cause of Imbalance lists to guide many of your questions by inquiring about things such as what season the condition began, what time of day it is better or worse, how old the person is, and so on. So if someone has say, upper respiratory mucous (catarrh), and it began in the winter time and is worse in the morning, it is pretty clear that you have agitated Water element. Of course, not everything will be this simple, but this gives you the idea.

Asking about Daily Habits is also important, as knowing how well someone is sleeping, what positions and physical actions dominate their day, what foods they eat, and what kind of exercises they engage in will all help to provide clues as to what may be amiss, and what may be causing it.

Sight

We use our sense of sight to visually assess the person we wish to help. Look at skin tone, physical posture, clearness of eyes, coloring, physical shape, and outward signs such as acne, rashes, flushing, and bruises. You can also look for signs of sweating, trembling, restlessness, and any other physical manifestations that can be seen with the naked eye. This is also inclusive of tongue and all other visual diagnostics, such as looking at the skin, eyes, nails, feces, urine, and any other visual inspection

Smell

With our sense of smell we can notice if someone has foul breath that might be indicative of digestive issues or oral/dental issues, we can assess toxic or stress sweat scents, and we can smell infection and yeasts. If we happen to have the chance to enter a bathroom after the patient, there are things that can be learned from the smell of their urine or feces that will be discussed later in this chapter. Smell can tell us if people smoke or drink to excess, as well as revealing certain diseases and stages of dying. The sense of smell is used to diagnose the urine, breath, feces, and body. Monitoring your own daily scents with awareness of your health is a good way to start getting proficient at understanding smells.

Touch

Palpation reveals if the skin is dry, oily, damp, hot, cold, thin, or thick—all of which are clues regarding elemental status. Touch can reveal hard-to-see swelling, inflammation, and conditions such as the tough or bumpy skin sometimes created by fungi. Going deeper, palpation can reveal adhesions, fatty deposits, tumors, quality of blood circulation, hydration of tissue and blood, and restriction in tissue, sên, and joints. As our sense of touch heightens and refines, we learn to sense areas that lack vitality in the body or are disconnected and becoming island "dead" zones.

Taste

In modern times the sense of taste is not often employed, but in times past doctors would use taste to detect clues from the patient's urine. While this may be unappealing, until recently it was generally accepted, even in the Western scientific community, that urine is usually sterile. This has been brought into doubt by recent studies, however. The degree of danger in ingesting urine is not currently known, and it is assumed to be relatively low. Regardless, most health care practitioners skip this part of Five Sense Diagnosis.

Digestive Diagnosis

In Traditional Thai Medicine, the primary focus when assessing a condition or looking at the general health of a patient is on diet, digestion, and elimination. So what we eat, how it's processed, and what it looks like when it comes out as feces are all important clues to ascertain what is going on. These things—new food, food in the stomach or small intestine, and feces—tell us a lot about health, and patients should be questioned about them anytime that internal balance is in doubt.

New Food
Ù-tá-rí-yá | อุทริยะ

What a person eats and craves can be a good indicator to their constitution, possible causes of imbalance, and assessing their imbalance. Is the person eating a lot of warming foods, such as peppery spicy flavors? Do they eat a lot of heavy, dense, damp food, such as pasta, oatmeal, and sweets? Do they eat lightly, snacking on small meals, fasting a lot, and easily skipping meals?

Food in the Stomach and Small Intestine

The success of the digestive process is down to the Fire element. If digestive fire is too strong, food will be broken down too fast, not giving the body a chance to absorb nutrients. It will pass through quickly, and there will likely be too much stomach acid or bile, with resulting problems from these fiery secretions. If digestive Fire is too weak, food will not break down and will sit in the upper digestive tract fermenting. This will result in accumulation of Wind in the form of gas, possibly creating bloating, belching, and passing gas. Food fermenting inside the digestive system also causes an accumulation of toxins in the body that can cause inflammation, illness, and pain.

Old Food/Feces
Gà-rì-sà | กรีส

We can learn a lot about how the body is functioning, as well as how well nutrients are being assimilated, by observing the stools, or feces, the quality, color and smell of which are good indicators of both major and minor imbalances. Be sure to keep in mind that it is important to know what a person has eaten recently, as this can lead to false diagnosis. For instance, beets will color feces red, which does not indicate a problem; iron supplements can cause black stools; and coffee can cause a fishy smell. Healthy stools are solid, not broken up, medium-brown colored, and the consistency of a ripe but not overripe banana (see? Thai medicine is so much fun!).

Old Food Color Indicators		
Element	Color	Explanation
Earth Imbalance	Feces will have a blackish coloring	Black feces are a result of digested blood, meaning that there is bleeding in the upper section of the digestive tract due to things such as lesions or sores in the stomach or small intestine. It can also indicate abnormalities in the spleen or liver. Again, Earth imbalance is generally indicative of more serious conditions. Black stools can also indicate that the liver is working too hard.
Water Imbalance	Feces will have a reddish coloring	Red generally indicates blood in the feces from the lower digestive tract. Often this is due to a lack of Water resulting in dryness, lack of lubrication causing abrasive feces passage.
Fire Imbalance	Feces will have a green or yellowish coloring	Green or very yellow feces indicates and excess of bile, or Fire, in the digestive system.
Wind Imbalance	Feces will have a white coloring	White, or light colored feces indicates mucous in the feces due to a lack of Wind and downward movement resulting in fermentation in the intestines and toxin formation. This irritates the mucous membrane and causes excessive mucous. Light color can also indicate that food is not absorbing well. Light colored stools can also indicate a deficient liver, blood deficiency, or too much Water.
Notes	If there is bleeding in the lower digestive tract, the feces will have actual blood in them.	

Old Food Scent Indicators		
Element	Smell	Explanation
Earth Imbalance	Feces have the smell of a decaying corpse	This is a terrible smell of course, and indicates serious imbalance such as cancer or infection of the tissue.
Water Imbalance	Feces have the smell of rotten fish	The rotten fish smell is a result of a bacterial infection. It is usually a lack of Fire that causes this, as the food is not digesting properly.
Fire Imbalance	Feces have the smell of burnt grass	The burnt grass smell comes from excessive Fire that burns the food.
Wind Imbalance	Feces have the smell of spoiled rice	The scent of spoiled rice indicates that feces are not being expelled from the body at a proper rate due to lack of Wind. They ferment in the colon.

Pulse Diagnosis

jàp chêep-pá-jon | จับชีพจร

Pulse diagnosis, whereby a doctor determines states of health by feeling the patient's pulses, can be found in traditional medicine all over the world. It is an extremely effective technique, but can take many years to master and should always be paired with other diagnostics. It is possible to use pulse diagnosis to ascertain a patient's core elemental constitution, current imbalance, and mental and physical conditions. Pulse diagnosis can be refined to the point where the condition of individual organs and systems in the body may be assessed. It is recommended that to truly learn pulse diagnosis you do not rely solely on a book but also seek out a qualified instructor, and make sure that you allow yourself years of touching as many pulses as you can before you expect proficiency.

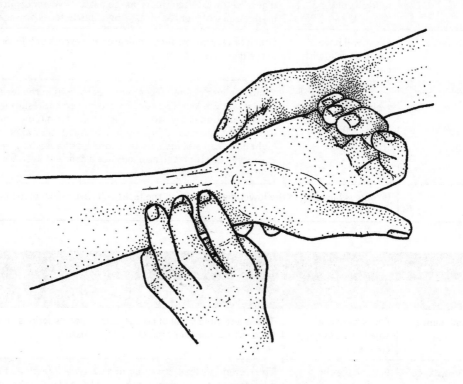

Pulse is the key diagnostic system of Traditional Thai Medicine. Currently, the Thai government is promoting a different diagnostic system, which is leading some to believe that pulse diagnosis is not a part of Thai medicine. Rest assured that it is not only a part of Traditional Thai Medicine but has its own methods that may be similar to, yet remain distinct from, Ayurvedic and Chinese pulse diagnostic systems.

Pulse is the preferred way of diagnosing elemental states because blood contains all of the elements. This is seen with the movement of blood being Wind element, the temperature of blood being Fire element, and the viscosity of blood being Water element. The particulates in blood are Earth element; however, in pulse diagnosis we focus on the more malleable three elements of Wind, Fire, and Water. Pulse diagnosis can give information about the whole body because the blood flows everywhere and communicates between the tissues. It connects one portion of the body to another as it travels throughout the body.

There are several different types of pulse diagnosis:

- *General Pulse Diagnosis* - This is used to get a sense of overall well-being.
- *Constitutional Pulse Diagnosis* - This is used to determine the individual's core elemental constitution.
- *Imbalance Pulse Diagnosis* - This is used to differentiate among the elements, determining which is strong, weak, predominant, and so on.
- *Organ or System Pulse Diagnosis* - This is used to tune in to specific organs and organ systems to determine their state of health. Here we can see, for example, if there is too much Fire in the spleen or if the stomach is too cold.

This book provides an overview of a general pulse diagnosis, as to study pulses in any depth requires an in-person teacher for adequate instruction. Pulses can be felt in various places around the body—primarily at the ankles, posterior knees, inguinal region, abdomen, neck, auxiliary region, elbows, and wrists. These places, where the pulse is easily felt, are called the Wind Gates. The best place to feel for pulse diagnostics is the wrist. This is because the wrists in a neutral position are central on the body, the pulse is easily felt here, and strong pressure can be applied without causing injury.

Ideally, pulse diagnosis of all kinds is done with the following conditions:

- In the morning
- Before the patient has eaten or had caffeine or cigarettes
- When the patient has not had sexual activity in the last 24 hours
- After the patient's bowels have been evacuated
- When the patient has not showered
- When no oil is on the patient's head or body for 24 hours
- When no exercise or heavy physical activity has been engaged in in the last 24 hours
- Minimal emotional disturbance (anger, joy, and so on)
- No alcohol or drugs in the last 24 hours.

Of course, these conditions can be very hard to meet, but if planning ahead to do pulse readings, do your best to observe these parameters. When you are unable to control for these factors, then keep them in mind while doing pulse reading. Remember that intense experiences such as strong emotions, exercise, and sex can have a significant impact on our pulses.

General Pulse Diagnosis

It's best to begin with doing the General Pulse Diagnosis. This will teach you the positioning for all the pulse diagnostic techniques, with the exception of the Body Diagnostic Pulse. It's also a good one for simply getting in touch with feeling pulses. As you begin to play with pulse diagnosis, remember to use all of your other diagnostic tools. Ask lots of questions. Pulse taking is not a parlor trick, in which you show what you can glean magically from touch alone. Even experienced doctors still do intakes. When you are first learning, asking questions is how you learn.

Characteristics of the Pulse

Before you begin taking pulses, read over the characteristics of the pulses. Then when you begin practicing, try to notice which of the characteristics are presenting. The more pulses you feel, the more clear these will become.

Pulse General Characteristics		
Fast or slow	Full or empty	Deep or Superficial
Large or Small	Steady or Uneven	Strong or Weak
Tense (hard) or Lax (soft)	Hot or Cold	Bounding

Pulse Element Characteristics	
Wind	Wind pulses are fast, feeble, cold, light, thin, weak, and disappear with pressure. They are felt under the index finger and move like a snake or a flag. Some texts say that Wind feels like an insect, being rapid.
Fire	Fire pulses are prominent, strong, have a high amplitude, are hot, forceful, and push up. They are felt under the middle finger and move like a frog or a chicken, jumping solidly and regularly.
Water	Water pulses are deep, slow, broad, wavy, thick, cool and regular. They are felt under the ring finger and move like a swan or an elephant. Water pulses are sluggish.

Positioning

The therapist and the patient should sit on the floor with legs crossed or in chairs, facing one another, and the therapist's eyes should be closed or unfocused, trained on the patient's forehead. Note: If sitting in chairs, do not cross the legs. The therapist holds the patient's hand gently with his or her nondominant hand, patient's hand is palm up, at the level of the patient's heart, with the patient's arm relaxed. The therapist's dominant hand will be the one actively feeling for the pulse. Traditionally, the right hand was always used to feel the pulse; however, this was most likely connected to general taboos against the left hand that stemmed from bathroom practices of using the left hand to clean oneself. Since the modern Western world does not have these practices or taboos, the left hand may be used; in fact, it may be the better hand for this purpose, as the left side is the "receiving" side of the body and is generally more attuned to sensory input. There should not be any more contact between the therapist and the patient than is necessary.

The therapist uses his or her index, middle, and ring fingers to feel for the pulse, with the index finger placed just proximal to the radial tuberosity in the soft trench just lateral of the center of the wrist. This is the Wind pulse position, and the index finger is the Wind finger when in a receiving action. The middle finger, which is the Fire finger when receiving, should be the distance of one grain of rice above the index finger. This is the Fire pulse position. And the ring finger, which is the Water finger when receiving, should be the width of one grain of rice above the middle finger, in the Water pulse position.

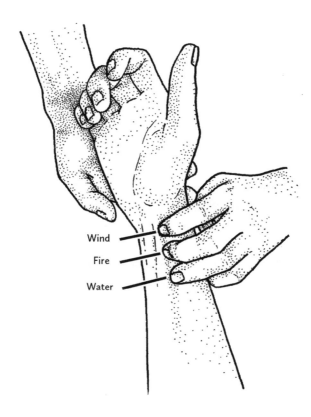

The reason that the different elements are felt in these spots has to do with the relative weight of the elements. Water, being the heaviest of the three, sinks down the deepest, and so must be felt closer to the heart. Wind, being the lightest, stays more superficial and may be felt the farthest from the heart. And Fire rests in the middle.

If checking the pulses at different places on the body, this arrangement remains the same, with the Water pulse always being closest to the heart. The different weight of the elements also gives us a clue as to the depth at which our fingers should rest. The ring finger will need to be ever so slightly deeper in order to reach the Water pulse, while the index finger will rest the most superficially. These distinctions are very slight, however; do not create a dramatic pressure difference between the fingers.

The parts of the fingers that make contact with the wrist should be the pads of the fingers. This is not the fingertips, but the little teardrop shaped pad that poofs out a bit on the underside of the last finger digit.

Some of the Traditional Thai Medicine texts say to take the pulse for men on the right, and women on the left; however, my teacher recommends doing both sides for each gender.

Method
- Sit in front of the patient.
- Hold the patient's hand with one hand and palpate the pulse with the other. Stare only at the center of the patient's forehead, or close the eyes.
- Apply gentle, steady pressure with your three pulse-feeling finger pads, feeling the pulse for at least thirty seconds. Relax your pressure for a rest moment, then palpate again the same way. Do this three times.
- Maintain full focus on the pulse and the patient the whole time, keeping out all distractions and not moving or talking. Try to allow yourself to be intuitive, and refrain from judgments. Have in mind the variables of age, season, and time.
- During this time you are experiencing and observing the pulses, noticing the characteristics that are present. Is the pulse strong? Weak? Bounding? Is it hot or cold? Is it displaying Wind characteristics of speed and slipperiness? Or is it hot and pounding into your fingers? Is it full and slow and cool like Water? Try to feel what is happening separately under each finger. Here, you are simply making contact with all three pulses, getting familiar with them. Do this on both the left and the right wrist. Begin to formulate an understanding of the messages the pulses are sending you, creating a generalized picture and getting an idea of how the elements are behaving.

Tongue Diagnosis

Tongue diagnosis in Thai medicine is primarily focused on digestive health, and to some degree the health of the heart and mind. Tongues are excellent for showing what is currently going on, as they have a very fast reaction time. If you are windy today, it shows on your tongue today. If you purge your body of toxins tomorrow, your tongue will show the purge tomorrow or the next day. The tongue is an almost immediate window into health.

A healthy tongue has medium thickness, a rounded front, a pink to reddish-pink coloring, and when pushed out of the mouth it holds itself in place without shaking or trembling. Unless otherwise noted, the following pathologies relate to the digestive system, specifically the part of the digestive system indicated by the map of the tongue. If a symptom shows on the entire tongue, it reveals a problem throughout the digestive system. It should be noted that any coating at all on the tongue indicates toxin formation and accumulation.

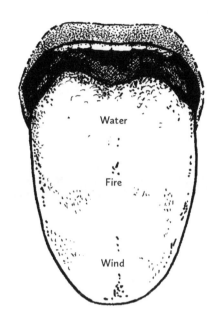
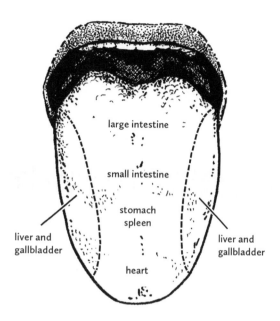

Color of Tongue			Coating of Tongue	
Pink/Reddish Pink	Healthy	White	Mucous that forms with depletion of Fire and Wind. Indicates regular toxins from eating bad foods and not digesting well.	
Light Pink	Deficiency/ too cold	Grey	Indicates Wind imbalance.	
White	Cold, damp, slow digestion	Brown	Indicates toxins caused by things rotting in the body. The blood will become toxic and poisoned to some degree. But be careful, it can also indicate that someone has been drinking coffee.	
Pale	Lack of Fire	Yellow	Shows excessive heat in the liver. This is often seen in people who have a fever.	
Dark / Bright Red	Heat in digestive system, too much Fire	Black	Indicates a serious problem such as black lungs and carcinogens. Black indicates that the pathology is affecting Earth element.	
Blue	Extreme cold, dampness			

Other Tongue Indicators	
Scalloped Edges	Indicates dampness, and a lack of nutrient absorption. Usually connected to weak Fire, but sometimes due to excess Wind moving food through the digestive system too fast.
Cracks	Indicates a weakness in the tissue (Earth) walls of the digestive system, or can indicate Wind issues.
Bumps	Often indicates lesions, polyps or ulcerations
Puffy Tongue	Indicates an excess of Water in the system. Can also point to a heaviness of mind
Dryness	Indicates a Wind imbalance.

What Tongues Tells us About The Mind	
Weak Tongue	Indicates a dull mind
Sharp Tongue (pointy sharp shape)	Indicates an alert and sharp mind, but often critical of others
Shaky Tongue	Indicates nervousness, agitated Wind imbalance or anxiety
Thick and Heavy Tongue	Indicates too much Water, and a sluggish or dull mind

Regarding coating, the tongue can be coated but dry, or coated and slippery. This shows the amount of Water in the body. If it has a mucous cover, or a stickiness to it, this shows excess Water. If the tongue is dry, whether or not it is coated, this shows deficient Water. If the coating is chunky or frothy, this shows dampness and excess Water. Scraping the coating off the tongue with a spoon or tongue scraper is beneficial, as the coating is a toxin waste product and this assists in removing it from the body.

Other Diagnostic Markers

Any part of the body may be looked at for clues as to what is ailing a person, but some are checked more frequently for specific pathologies, such as the tongue being looked at for the digestive system and the mind. Here are a smattering of other diagnostic markers.

Eyes

Place your finger just under the lower lid, and gently tug the tissue down so that the inner lip of the lower eyelid shows. Check for paleness or redness. Paleness indicates depletion and low vitality, while bright or dark redness indicates too much heat in the blood, as eyes show the temperature of the blood. If the liver is being affected by excessive heat the color will be yellowish. If it has a gray quality to it, then Wind is imbalanced.

Skin

Dry skin indicates excess Wind, damp skin shows excess Water, and oily skin reveals excess Fire.

Face

The shape of the face is an indicator of the core elemental constitution. If the face is wider toward the top, Wind dominates. If it is wider near the middle (around eye level), then Fire is dominant. And if the face is wide toward the lower third of the face, then Water element dominates.

Nails

As with the lower eyelid, nails are used an indicator of the temperature of the body and to check for circulation. Look at the nails for the color underneath. It should be a light pink. White shows a lack of circulation, bluish-gray shows a Wind imbalance, and bright red shows a Fire imbalance. Press down on the nail, hold a moment, then release. Watch to see how quickly the color returns. If the color returns slowly, then circulation is poor.

Menses

A woman's menstrual cycle tells a Traditional Thai Medicine practitioner many things. It is normal for a Thai medicine doctor to ask female patients for detailed descriptions of their cycle.

Menstruation Indicators	
Wind Imbalance	Pre-menstrual gas and nausea, possible fevers. Flow may be uneven, foamy and dark
Fire Imbalance	Pre-menstrual skin irritation. Temperature swings between hot and cold. Blood may be bright red, or yellow.
Water Imbalance	Pre-menstrual stomach aches and diarrhea, with depleted appetite. Blood will be clear and mucousy
Earth Imbalance	Pre-menstrual joint and bone pain. Stomach aches and dark red blood with a strong odor.
Toxic Blood	Irregular painful menses, dark and chunky blood, strong body and breath odor with periods.

Spirit Diagnosis

Problems with the spirit world are found through the same diagnostic process as any other disorder, using intake, palpation, divination, and examination. Generally if no other source of the problem is found, it is assumed to be an issue involving ghosts, spirits, kwǎn, or deities.

Divinatory Diagnosis

The oracular root of Thai medicine incorporates usage of many divinatory sciences to ascertain ailments that are likely to manifest in the future, or are currently present. These include astrology, numerology, palmistry, geomancy, and other more esoteric forms of divination, many of which are based in a variety of mathematical calculations.

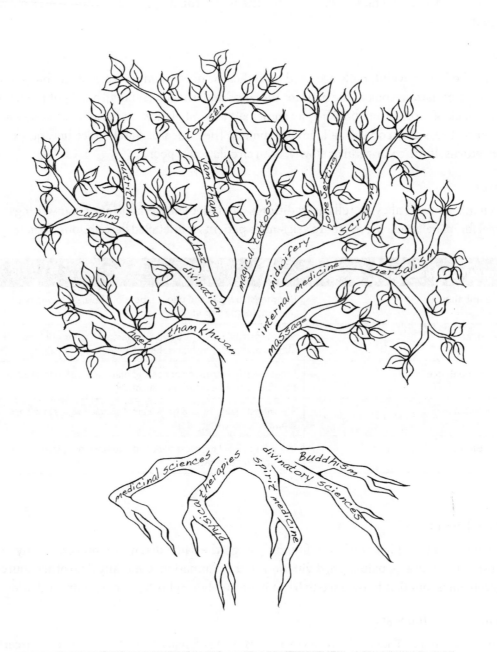

PART 2

The Roots of Thai Medicine

AS WE LEAVE BEHIND DISEASE CAUSATION and diagnosis and wade into the bones of therapies, we will engage with the five roots of Thai medicine primarily, but not exclusively, with bodyworkers in mind. There will, however, be teachings that do not seem on the surface to apply to a bodywork practice. We will talk a bit about herbal medicine and ghosts and the teachings of the Buddha. This is because the tradition of learning Thai medicine does not segregate its component parts the way that Western medicine does. There is much overlap between roots, specialties, and practices, and honestly, there is stuff I want to tell you about that just might not hold to the parameters of a massage practice—because, well, it's just good stuff.

Also, it must be understood that regardless of your medical specialty, a basic understanding of all the roots of Thai medicine is required. For instance, a midwife must know medical theory, herbal medicine, massage, and other forms of physical therapy to help the mother. She must also understand astrology and spirits in order to help prevent any negative influences upon the mother and child, and she must have a foundation in Buddhism to be able to help counsel her patients should things such as child death occur.

The five roots are the basis of, and integral to, all medical specialties, whether you are a medical doctor, pharmacist, massage therapist, midwife, spirit/witch doctor, astrologer, or herbalist. These are the roots that form the entire tree of Thai medicine, and no part, no branch or leaf, exists that isn't connected through the trunk to all five roots.

Roots of Traditional Thai Medicine			
English	**Thai Phonetic**	**Thai Breakdown**	**The Practice**
1. Medicinal Sciences Internal therapies, herbalism	แพทยศาสตร์ *Pâet sàat*	*Pâet* = medicine, a doctor, drugs, etc. *Sàat* = knowledge, study, science	Preparation and (internal and external) administration of medicines including plants, minerals and animals in the form of single herb medicines, compound herb medicines, and use of food as medicine.
2. Physical Therapies Orthopedic medicine, External therapies	กายภบำบัด *Gaai-yá bam-bàt*	*Gaai-yá* = body, physical *Bam-bàt* = therapy	All physical therapies applied to the external body.
3. Divination Oracular sciences	โหราศาสตร์ *Hŏh raa sàat*	*Hŏh raa* = an astrological chart *Sàat* = knowledge, study, science	Use of systems such as astrology, numerology, palmistry, geomancy, tarot and other oracular sciences to determine health of body mind and spirit.
4. Spirit Medicine Magical, spirit practices	ไสยศาสตร์ *Săi-yá-sàat*	*Săi-yá-* = magic *Sàat* = knowledge, study, science	Use of spirits, amulets, incantations, magical tattoos, spiritual herbalism, demons, deities and other practices for healing arts, protection and attraction.
5. Buddhism Mental health & harmonious living	พุทธศาสตร์ *Pút-tá-sàat*	*Pút-tá* = the Thai pronunciation of the word Buddha *Sàat* = knowledge, study, science	Understanding suffering and how to ease suffering through the dharma.

A couple of things about translations should be mentioned here. At first I called the medicinal sciences root "Herbalism." This is close but not as exact as medicinal sciences, as the word herbalism doesn't cover the full scope of this root. However, in discussing this root in the following chapter, I have primarily stuck with the herbalism aspect of it as this is quite applicable to a bodywork practice.

Also, in relation to the Orthopedic Medicine root, there has been some debate in Western Thai massage circles about using words like "bodywork" to describe Thai massage. Somehow there has been confusion in which some people have come to think that Thai massage falls under the heading of "energy work," and that terms that elicit thoughts of stronger physicality are incorrect. However, if you look to the root that massage branches from, we see that the literal translation of *Gaai-yá-bam-bàt* is physical, or body, therapies. A more accurate term than "Thai massage" would be "Thai physical therapies." It is, inherently, a deeply physical healing art.

Of course, Thai medicine has many aspects that are more focused on less physically intensive therapies, but most of these are from the Spirit Medicine, Divinatory Sciences, and Buddhism roots.

Another translation that bears mentioning is Spirit Medicine. The more precise translation of *Săi-yá-sàat* would be Magical Sciences; however, I decided to go with Spirit Medicine in order to avoid confusion and visions of stage theatrics with disappearing rabbits. From the Five Roots of Thai Medicine, many healing arts specialties arise. The following chart shows some of the main ones, each of which may have a variety of subspecialties.

Traditional Thai Medicine Specialties		
Herbal Medicine ยาสมุนไพร *Yaa sà-mŭn prai or yaa môr* ยาหม้อ This is internal herbal medicine as well as dietary and lifestyle adjusting	**Midwifery** ผดุงครรภ์ *Pà-dung kan* Pre and post natal care. Midwifery employs much bodywork, spirit work, and herbalism	**Massage** นวด *Nûat* Inclusive of many external body therapies, including many specialties listed in this chart plus and more.
Nutritional Counseling โภชนาการ *poh-chá-naa gaan* Dietetics for elemental balance and general health	**Divination** หมอดู *mŏr doo* Including astrology, geomancy, numerology, tarot and palmistry	**Bone setting** จัดกระดูก *jàt grà-dòok* Includes the setting of broken bones, and also all indigenous chiropractics
Spirit Doctors หมอผี *mŏr pĕe* Uses incantations, amulets, and works with spirits.	**Magical Tattooing** สักยันต์ *sàk yan* Sacred words and symbols tattooed on the body.	**Herbal Compresses** ลูกประคบ *lôok bprà-kóp* Use of herbs on the external body.
Point Work กดจุด *gòt jùt* Acupressure on release points **Cupping** แก้วสูญญากาศ *gâew sŏon-yaa-gàat* Use of suction to draw out toxins and heat	**Tok Sên** ตอกเส้น *does not have an English name* Percussive therapy combining use of tools and spirit medicine. Tok sên has recently become popular as a simple massage modality being picked up by westerners, however it is not fully effective without proper initiation and training if one is following tradition.	**Yam kăng** ย่ำขาง *yam kăng* Spirit medicine that employs use the feet applied with oils and fire. These days being misinterpreted as a massage modality, however it doesn't work without Spirit Medicine training and initiations.
Chét and hâek เช็ดแฮก *does not have an English name* A spirit medicine technique that employs gently rubbing a sacred object on the patient while chanting incantations.	**Jòp kài** จอบไข่ *does not have an English name* Removal of toxins and evil with an egg. This is another spirit medicine technique.	**Bpào** เป่า *does not have an English name* Blowing sacred words. This is like Chét Hâek without the tool.
Scraping การครูด *gaan krôot* Use of tools to gently pull out toxins and heat by repetitive non abrasive scraping.	**Blood Letting** ผ่าเลือดออก *pàa lêuat òk* Generally localized release of stagnant or toxic blood. Sometimes systemic release.	**Nûat Karsai** นวด กระษัย Abdominal organ massage. These days being misinterpreted as massage specifically for reproductive organs; traditionally for all organs.

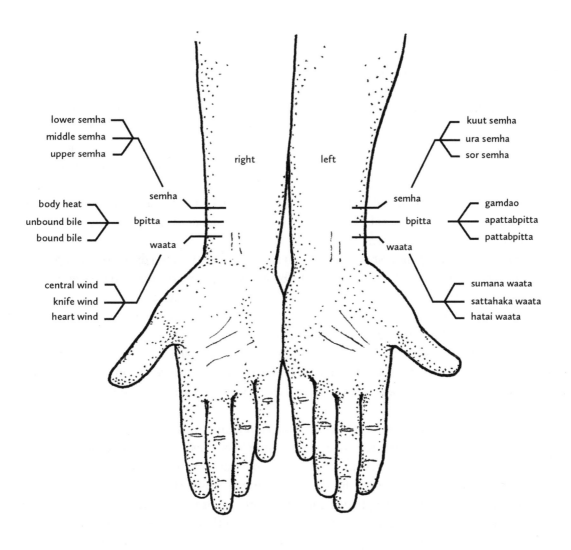

lower semha
middle semha
upper semha

right

left

kuut semha
ura semha
sor semha

body heat
unbound bile
bound bile

semha
bpitta
waata

semha
bpitta
waata

gamdao
apattabpitta
pattabpitta

central wind
knife wind
heart wind

sumana waata
sattahaka waata
hatai waata

CHAPTER FOUR

Thai Medicinal Science
Internal Medicine, Herbology, & General Medicine
Pâet sàat | แพทยศาสตร์

WHEN I FIRST STARTED studying Thai medicine with my teacher, my focus was entirely on bodywork. My teacher and I had several conversations that went like this:

Teacher: "Nephyr, read about this herb and know its tastes and what it's for." Me: "Um, okay, but I just do massage; I'm not an herbalist." Teacher: "Yes, I know. So, go read about this herb."

This conversation happened a lot. One day we were in Bangkok, and just before I flew home to the US, my teacher bought several little bags of herbs from an herb shop and gave them to me, with instructions to soak them in alcohol for three months, then remove some of the alcohol and set it aside and then add certain other herbs to the rest of the alcohol. He told me the set-aside alcohol was for internal use, "You know, like if someone is shot," and the rest was for external use on traumatic injuries.

I did not immediately understand that "like if someone is shot" was a dramatic example that meant it was good for all sorts of trauma to the body, including more common injuries such as sprains and strains, but eventually I caught on. I made the formulas, and at first they just sat around, barely on my radar. Then friends started getting hurt, and I started giving them these formulas—and watching the rapid recoveries with a bit of amazement.

A handful of months later, my teacher sent me a box full of Thai herbs and herbal products. To my inquiries about what some capsules full of green powder were for, my teacher wrote: "For if you get poisoned." Images of arsenic and castle intrigue floated through my head, and I put the capsules aside.

About a month later I went out with a dear friend, and I drank a glass of wine. Now at this time I had not had alcohol for about a year, simply because it's not something I tend to gravitate towards. I went home, went to bed, and about an hour later I woke up feeling horrible. As I lay in bed trying to assess how I felt, the only words that fit were "I feel poisoned." As soon as the words went through my head, I thought of those green capsules. Really, I knew nothing about them. I didn't know if they would help with an adverse reaction to alcohol, how many to take, or what to expect. But I trusted that my teacher would not have given me a dangerous herb without warnings, so I took two capsules and went back to bed. After twenty minutes lying in my bed, I quite clearly felt my blood washing clean. It was like a wave of clean water coursed through my body and all feelings of imbalance vanished. I have since used this herb to vanquish adverse reactions to MSG as well as to reduce fevers. Always with tangible results.

From that time on, I have had a growing love and understanding of Thai herbalism (as well as an appreciation for the extremes my teacher uses to describe the purpose of remedies). The observable effectiveness of the herbs and formulas never ceases to amaze me. I have written about Thai herbs more extensively[56] in *Thai Herbal Medicine: Traditional Recipes for Health and Harmony,* and I will refer readers to that book for more information and formulas so as not to be repetitive here, or simply for those who thirst to go more in depth with Thai herbalism.

Here, I will present the basic foundational information on Thai herbalism, as well as some of my favorite herbal remedies. I want to note, though, that while my focus here is herbs, this root of medicine is not all about herbs. It is inclusive of the preparation and administration of a wide variety of medicines made from everything from bones to minerals, as well as general medical diagnostics.

Tastes

Western herbalism categorizes herbs by function (i.e. anti-inflammatory, emetic, and antipyretic).[57] Thai herbalism, like Ayurvedic medicine, categorizes herbs by taste, wherein each herb is found to have a particular taste, and each taste has a particular effect on each element, being either nourishing, neutral, or calming to the element.

There are several taste systems in Thai medicine, with different ones being used for different purposes.

For instance, a nine-taste system is used when referring to single herbs being used as medicine, whereas a six-taste system is used when referring to herbs that are used in foods (since there are some tastes that are used medicinally that you would not want to put in dinner), and a four-taste system is used when talking about herbs used on the external body, such as in liniments and compresses. Additionally there is an eight-taste system used when speaking of herbs that serve as vehicles for other medicines (such as herbs that help the body to absorb the medicine or direct it to the right place in the body) as well as a three taste system that actually employs temperatures not tastes.

---

56 With my co-author of that book (and its original creator) Pierce Salguero.
57 Emetic = induces vomiting; Anti-Pyretic = reduces fever

Nine Taste System · *single herbs used medicinally*			
Astringent *rót fàat* รสฝาด	Binding, dries Water and heals wounds	**Oily** *rót man* รสมัน	Corrects the *sên*, lubricates the body, nourishes bone marrow and is a tonic for the tissue
Sweet *rót wǎan* รสหวาน	Permeating, nourishes tissue, treats malaise and strengthens	**Fragrant/Cool** *rót hǒm yen* รสหอมเย็น	Refreshes, calms mental Winds, eases stress, and is a heart mind tonic.
Toxic *rót mao bèua* รสเนาเบื่อ	Corrects poison, treats toxins and fever	**Salty** *rót kem* รสเค็ม	Permeates the skin, preserves tissue and treats skin diseases
Bitter *rót kǒm* รสขม	Corrects blood, reduces fever, tonic for blood and bile, and increases appetite	**Sour** *rót bprîeow* รสเปรี้ยว	Cuts mucous, expels toxins, purges, and cleans blood
Spicy/hot *rót pèt rón* รสเผ็ดร้อน	Corrects Wind, treats digestive Wind, moves menstrual blood and treats & tonifies the elements	**Tasteless** *rót jèut* รสจืด (tasteless makes this list ten, however, because it is tasteless, traditional teachings say nine tastes)	Corrects mucous, calms Fire including fever, supports kidneys, absorbs poison

More about these Tastes
Astringent = foods that leave a dry feeling in the mouth, such as unripe bananas or pomegranate skins
Sweet = all sweets of course, but if speaking of foods for health, think of natural sweets such as dates and honey
Intoxicating = herbs that introduce toxins to the body including mind altering substances, but also herbs that make you purge (vomiting, sweating, defecating...).
Bitter = herbs such as bitter greens and arugula
Spicy/hot = strong heating herb such as chilies and black or long pepper, but also gentle warming herbs such as cumin, coriander and cinnamon.
Oily = nuts, seeds and oils
Fragrant/cool = flowers such as jasmine and rose
Salty = salt of course, and salty herbs such as fish and celery
Sour = sour herbs such as lemons and limes.
Tasteless = any medicinal herb that lacks flavor, such as clay

When we speak of herbs in traditional medicine, the word is used for more than just plants; it covers anything you can ingest, including meats, oils, horns, insects, and minerals.

Six Taste System · *herbs used in food*			
Bitter (Very cooling)	Increases or nourishes Wind, Calms Water and Fire	**Salty** (Mildly warming)	Increases or nourishes Water and Fire, Calms Wind
Spicy/Hot (Very warming)	Increases or nourishes Fire, Calms Water	**Sour** (Moderately warming)	Increases or nourishes Water and Fire, Calms Wind
Astringent (Moderately cooling)	Increases or nourishes Wind, Calms Fire and Water	**Sweet** (Mildly cooling)	Increases or nourishes Water, Calms Fire and Wind

The charts of the nine- and six-herb taste systems is to help you with understanding food and herb recommendations that may appear in this book, but is a very basic overview. For more in-depth understanding of these systems, as well as an extensive herbal compendium, refer to the book *Thai Herbal Medicine*.

Four-Taste System for the External Body

The four-taste system and the three-taste system are the taste systems that most apply to a bodywork practice. The four-taste system is based on tastes that penetrate the first four layers of the body via application of herbs to the skin (organs must be reached through internal ingestion of herbs).

Spicy/Hot

Herbs that fall in this category, such as chilies, onions, long pepper, black pepper, camphor, and garlic, penetrate the layer of the skin. They remove stagnation through heat and relieve pain. They also open this layer of the body, allowing for sweat to remove toxins from the body and allowing herbs to penetrate the deeper layers. For this reason, herbal formulas meant for the tissue, *sên*, or bone layers will usually have some spicy/hot herbs in them. Do not use heating herbs in instances of rashes, inflammation, or fever.

A subcategory of Spicy/Hot is Aromatic/Pungent. These are warming herbs that are not spicy, such as nutmeg, lemongrass, cinnamon (also sweet), and *plai* (also astringent). Camphor and borneol—hot and aromatic pungent, respectively—are herbs that have a special ability to transport other herbs through the skin layer and are often found in Thai herbal formulas for physical therapies.

Astringent

Astringent herbs permeate the three layers of the skin as well as just to the tissue. This is really around the superficial fascia, between the deepest layer of skin and tissue. Astringent assists in wound healing, drying out dampness, and drawing out toxins. Herbs such as turmeric, green tea, and *plai* are examples of astringent. Astringent herbs have a unique ability to dry out and knit, or bind, tissue, making them very good for wounds. Of course, because of this they are not beneficial to those with dehydrated skin and tissue.

Sour

Sour taste is very important because it benefits the muscles and also works on the *sên*. Herbs such as kaffir lime skin, tamarind, and senna penetrate to the tissue and the *sên*, where they purge blockages, clear the channels, and move Wind. Most internal purgatives have sour taste in them. Applied externally, it essentially does the same thing in terms of moving out what is stuck. Sour should not be used excessively as it can putrefy the tissue.

Salty

Here, we are usually straight up talking about sea salt or rock salt. Salt permeates to the bone and softens hardened tissue and masses, as well as healing adhesions. Almost all compresses have salt in them for the bones, and also because salt retains heat. Salt should not be used on an open wound or with pregnancy.

If you look at the ingredients in most Thai herbal compresses, balms, liniments, poultices, and plasters, you will find that they are often a mixture of herbs from these taste categories. Understanding the role of the different tastes can be beneficial in creating your own formulas, and provides deeper understanding about what the products you are using are for. The four tastes presented above are listed in traditional medicine texts, but practically speaking, sweet and bitter tastes are also used in the external application of herbs.

Sweet

Sweet works on the tissue layer, permeating to the muscle and the fat. It is very nourishing for the tissue and sedates and calms the nerves that exist on this layer as well. Sweet is used in the form of oil in liniments and balms. In this instance, we are not talking about sugar, but rather a mellower quality of sweet, such as is found in oils and certain herbs.

Bitter

Bitter works on the blood and the channels. It purifies and maintains smooth flow of the blood and also maintains a richness to it. Bitter is important for inflammatory conditions such as boils and inflammation from injury.

Three-Temperature System

The three-taste system isn't really about tastes; rather, it refers to temperatures. All other herbal medicines and products can be understood through this system, and it becomes a simplified approach to medicine. By understanding if a condition would benefit most from heating therapies, mild/neutral therapies, or cooling therapies, you can navigate much of Thai medicine. Heating and cooling herbs and formulas are on a spectrum, with neutral in the middle. So while two formulas may both be heating, they are not necessarily heating to the same degree. For instance, all sweet-tasting herbs are cool; however, honey is the warmest of the sweet herbs, falling closer to center yet still on the cool side of the spectrum.

Heating

Single herbs and formulas that heat the body, of course, fall into the heating category. Heating formulas treat gross Winds and some conditions of Water element, in particular accumulations of toxins and stagnation. Heating herbs assist movement, as seen with increased circulation (Fire excites Wind), movement freed via the relaxation of tense tissue through heating therapies, and the purging created through sweating. They are also very good for treating flatulence, indigestion, and general Wind in the digestive system.

In physical therapies, the external use of heating balms, liniments, and compresses assists with relaxing tissue, increasing circulation, removing stagnation, and nourishing depletion. Heating therapies are not recommended in cases of excited or excess Fire, including any toxic fever such as influenza or malaria. Be careful with heating formulas when there is heat or extreme conditions.

Cooling

Cooling herbs and formulas contain herbs that have cooling properties. They are used to calm the Fire element. Cooling herbs taken internally treat toxic fevers, subdue poison, treat excessive sweating or body heat, and help to regulate Fire element. Externally, they are beneficial for rashes, excess heat near the surface of the body, and traumatic injuries. Traditional medicine does not use ice in cases of acute injuries; rather, it uses cool water or herbs with cooling qualities. Do not use cooling herbs with Wind imbalances.

Mild/Neutral

Mild herbs are neither heating nor cooling. They are used to treat the subtle Winds (herbs like cardamom), to treat the blood, and to control excessive mucous. Internally, they are cleansing for the blood and treat mucous. Do not use mild herbs with toxic fevers, such as dengue fever, yellow fever and malaria. Traditional texts say that mild temperature treats Water element, but not if there are toxins and stagnation.

Regarding Local and Imported Herbs

A question that comes up a lot in my classes is: Aren't local herbs better for you? It's a valid and interesting question, to which there isn't a simple answer. There is certainly truth to the idea that we resonate with our environment and that which grows in it; yet, we have had a global spice trade for thousands of years, and there is no denying the medicinal effects of many imported herbs. If we agree that food is medicine, we can see that we have been medically nourishing ourselves with herbs from faraway places for a very long time. In the West, from black pepper to cinnamon, from ginger to cloves, we have been introducing these foreign herbs to our bodies for millennia. Still, some things, such as honey, are clearly more beneficial if locally harvested, and there is the environmental factor of export/import to consider. This is a book on Thai medicine, so the use of herbs that must travel the globe to reach you is inherent; but some can be found around the world, and I do encourage use of local sources whenever possible.

In order to imbue nonnative herbs with a local energetic, there are two things you can do. One is to find local nutgrass root, which grows all over the world, and make a tea of it. Drink this tea when ingesting foreign herbs medicinally. Nutgrass picks up the energetics of a particular region, climate, or season, and harmonizes whatever you are taking with that place. The second thing that you can do is to take locally harvested raw honey[58] with your medicine, as this will have the same effect.

A Bodyworker's Herb Basket

What follows here is some of those herbs, formulas, and products that are my favorites but which didn't make it into *A Thai Herbal*. (Note: I've left out of both books overly complex formulas, or those requiring herbs that you must travel to Thailand to purchase.)

Please keep in mind that anyone can have an allergic reaction to any herb in a formula. There is no such thing as a completely benign herb or food. I have met people with deathly serious allergies to everything from kiwis to tofu. Always make sure that patients who you wish to receive herbal formulas are aware of the ingredients in the formula and understand the potential risk of taking it. Any doubts or questions should be discussed with a trained herbalist or physician. Most of the time, measurements do not need to be exact, but try to come close. Unless very specific quantities are noted, a part is an amount of your choosing, but all parts should match. So whether you decide that one part is 2 ounces or 1 kilo, be sure to use this ratio for the whole formula.

Thai Herbal Compresses
lôok bprà-kóp | ลูกประคบ

Okay, these are simply the best things ever. For many years, I didn't use compresses because I thought they were a fluffy, spalike addendum to Thai massage—a pampering device, if you will. Not that there is anything wrong with pampering, but I've always gotten more pleasure out of doing the "fixit" kind of bodywork. How silly I was! If only I had known that Thai herbal compresses are the fixit to trump most fixits! They are pampering fixits! The most generic, packaged, pre-made compress has therapy value beyond some of my most beloved hands-on massage techniques. They calm the mental Winds with lovely scents, the herbal steam cleanses the sinuses and lungs, the heat relaxes the body and the herbs—well, what the herbs do depends on the kind of compress, but in general they heal and relax and release. And everyone, everyone, loves them.

To use hot herbal compresses, steam them for fifteen to thirty minutes,[59] wrap in a face towel, and gently press the compress to the body, rolling it away from you. Keep in touch with the massage recipient to find out if the compress is too hot (in which case press more gently and move more quickly until it cools a bit) or too cool (in which case exchange it for a fresh compress). When the compresses are still warm but not so hot as to risk burning, they can be pressed into the body fairly firmly, creating both a massage tool and a warming herbal treatment.

---

58 Being a long time vegan and lifelong vegetarian, I have sympathy for the bees that make our honey. A bee only makes about one-half teaspoon of honey in its entire life. That's a lot of work! I encourage thoughtful use of honey, and purchasing it from kind-hearted beekeepers who go to lengths to take good care of their bees, not smoking them out, or leaving them with crappy, overly processed sugar replacement for their honey. That said, at this point, bees and people have a bit of a symbiotic relationship going on, so the keeping of bees grows ever more important.

59 If the compresses are made of dried herbs, submerge them in water for about 10 seconds before steaming.

How to Make Thai Herbal Compresses

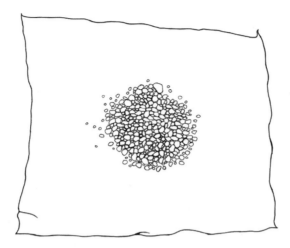

1. Chop herbs small and place about 2 cups of herbs in the center of a square cloth.

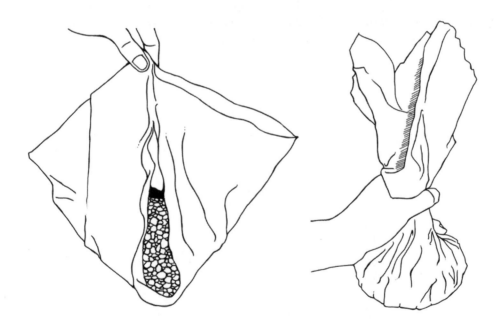

2. Gather the corners of the cloth together, and let the mid folds point out.

3. Twist the extra cloth beginning at the base above the herbs. Try to keep everything extremely tight.

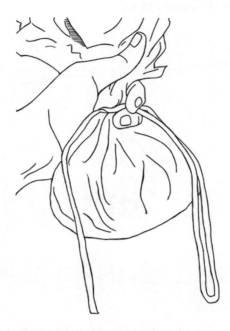

4. Loop a string around the base of the twist, leaving a short string tail, and then wrapping the longer side of the string up the twist to the top, and then back down to the base. The top of the twisted cloth can be folded over such that the string wraps it all up with no loose cloth. At the base, tie the remaining string to the tail.

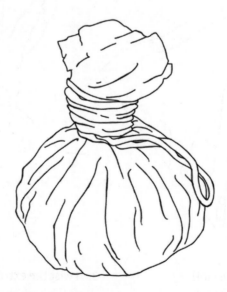

5. And *voilà!* You have a lovely Thai herbal compress!

Pre-made Warming Compress

Most of the generic, pre-made, dried Thai herbal compresses are warming. They all have similar but slightly different formulas, which are designed to help as many people as possible—kind of a catchall of herbal compresses. They contain herbs for all four layers of the body (excluding the fifth, the organs), and because most people experience tension, adhesions, and a variety of tissue layer aches and pains, they are warming. If you are buying pre-made compresses, test some out from different suppliers to find ones that you love. There are two traditional warming compress formulas given in *Thai Herbal Medicine*, if you wish to make them yourself.

Compress for Bruising, Blood, and Muscles

This compress can be adapted, depending on your focus, and for this reason I am providing a brief description of what each herb is good for. You can use the formula as given, or adjust the quantities as needed. Try to get as many of the herbs fresh as you can. This is mostly for blood and bruising. It will help draw out toxins and will move blood.

- Kaffir lime leaf
- Kaffir lime peel
- *Plai* (Cassumar ginger)
- Ginger
- Galanga
- Cinnamon
- Turmeric
- Rock salt
- Camphor

This is an adjustable formula. Regardless of how many of the other herbs you choose to use, only use a little bit of camphor (about one-half teaspoon per compress) and a moderate amount of salt. The Kaffir lime helps to draw out toxins and treat tendon and ligaments. The ginger and turmeric are good for the skin; cinnamon and galangal help to move the blood; salt aides the bones; and camphor is both for the mind and to help the other herbs to permeate. *Plai* is for bruising, blood, and muscles. If you cannot find *plai* you can omit it, however the formula is better with it. Chop or grind the herbs into rough, small pieces and follow basic compress-making instructions.

Simple Coconut Cooling Compress

Unsweetened dried shredded coconut with a little rock salt makes for a perfect cooling compress. Simply wrap in cloth, and steam for about fifteen minutes. Allow the compress to cool a little before using. It will still be warm, but with the purpose being to support the cooling quality of the coconut. Using it while it's very hot is counterproductive.

Prenatal Bodywork Compress

Thai prenatal massage is done almost entirely with herbal compresses, as is further detailed in the physical therapies section. Here is a lovely prenatal massage compress formula.

Equal parts:
- Mint
- Coriander
- Rose flowers
- Jasmine flowers
- Dried shredded coconut
- Turmeric
- Dried white rice

You can use dried or fresh herbs, but choose one and stick to it. Do not mix dried and fresh (with the exception of the rice and coconut, which will be dried in either case). Mix the ingredients together and bundle as tightly as you possibly can in cloth tied to make round compresses. It generally takes a lot more herbs than one thinks it will to make a tightly compacted compress. Steam the compresses for about fifteen minutes before removing one to work with.

Postpartum Bodywork Dry Compress

For postpartum massage you can use any generic pre-made Thai warming compress, or you can make these compresses that are specifically designed to assist with removing excess fluids from the body, including drying the uterus and encouraging the uterus to contract down to pre-pregnancy size. These are also beneficial for postpartum detoxification. Dry compresses are employed when the goal is to counter excess moisture in the body. These can be steamed, if necessary, but it is better to use the dry heat method provided in the notes below. The following formula makes one compress.

- 2 cups rock salt
- 3 dried nutmegs, loosely crushed
- 5 dried long peppers, loosely crushed
- 3 sticks dried cinnamon

Rock salt can be purchased in most grocery stores, where it is usually sold for making ice cream. To make this compress, place the mixture of salt and herbs in a dry cast iron or stainless steel skillet over medium high heat and stir while heating. Once the salt and herbs are quite hot, pour into a cloth bag, a clean sock, or any cloth vessel. Use as you would use steamed compresses to massage the body. When the compress cools, pour the herbs back in the skillet and reheat. Repeat process to massage with the compress again, at least five times. Alternatively, this mixture can be made into compresses as normal, and heated in an oven; however, you must wet the cloth to prevent burning, and it can be tricky to get the temperature just right.

The reason for using forms of dry heat such as the skillet or the oven, as opposed to steaming is that you want to dry out the postpartum tissue and uterus, so introducing the wetness of steam would be counterproductive. These compresses are contraindicated for pregnancy and should only be used postpartum.

Liniments, Balms and Poultices

Get a Thai massage in Thailand, and chances are high that you will leave with some part of your body feeling icy hot and smelling like a whole mess of aromatic herbs. This is because they use herbal balms and liniments extensively in Thai bodywork. We tend to know about this side of Thai medicine through Tiger Balm™, a mass-produced Thai herbal balm. Just about any Thai herbalist you meet in Thailand will have their own formula for balms and liniments, and most people who do bodywork keep a good stock of them around. These products are used primarily for spot-specific treatment of aches, pains, tension, injury, and many other specific ailments.

When you use balms and liniments in bodywork, remember that the goal is to get the herbs into the body. Don't just lightly slap on some liniment and leave it at that. No, you need to really massage it into the skin and tissue. Once it is absorbed, then apply some more, and massage that in, too. If someone has something wrong that you feel will benefit greatly from a balm or a liniment that you have, it's best to send them home with some and give instructions for it to be applied several times a day. This sort of serious approach to the use of balms and liniments is what will give them a chance to be of most benefit.

Regarding Oils

Oils often have healing properties all by themselves and can serve as a simple liniment. When buying oil, try to find oil that is raw, unfractionated, and unrefined. Coconut oil should smell like coconut, and sesame oil should not smell toasted.

COCONUT OIL is on the cooler side. It is beneficial for the skin and aids sore and achy muscles. It also helps to penetrate the skin layer and can soothe sunburns and dry, cracked skin.

RAW SESAME OIL is a much warmer oil. It doesn't have the properties of relieving muscular pain, but it is good for gently warming the body, and it is the best carrier for herbs. Raw sesame oil is beneficial for those with excited Wind element who tend to run cold. It can be rubbed on the body once or twice a day to ground, warm, and soothe.

SAFFLOWER OIL is somewhere in between coconut and sesame oil in temperature, and is a good tonic for the skin. It is often used instead of sesame oil, or mixed with sesame oil, simply because it is less expensive.

Drawing Liniment

This liniment draws toxic blood and stagnation from the deeper levels, dispersing it and drawing it out through the skin. It is especially good to use when cupping and scraping show toxins through dark discoloration; it is also beneficial for bruises, especially deep bruises. This liniment reaches to the layer of the *sên,* where the herbs dissipate stagnation and the castor oil draws it to the surface. This is a very viscous formula, which is applied at the end of a treatment. A good drawing liniment belongs in every bodyworker's tool basket.

Approximately half a cup of each herb:
- Long pepper
- Cinnamon
- Clove
- Safflower
- Black pepper
- Frankincense
- Calamus
- Sesame and/or safflower oil (all sesame is best, but quite expensive, so you can either cut it 50/50 with safflower oil, or replace it altogether with safflower oil if necessary)
- Castor oil [60]

Pulverize all the herbs in a mortar and pestle under they are close to powder in consistency. If you use a coffee grinder you must pulse it and be very careful not to let it get too hot, as heat will change the properties of the herbs. Put the herbs in a glass jar, and add sesame and/or safflower oil, enough to make a thick paste. Then add about one inch more oil that floats on top of the paste and mix it in. Cover with plastic wrap and a lid. Leave overnight, and check the next day; the herbs will have settled and the oil should be one inch above them; if it's not, add more oil. Let sit for twelve days wrapped in a thick paper bag in a warm place, turning it daily. You can put it on a water heater or in the sun, but it must be dark (hence the bag). After twelve days, strain out the herbs, then heat over very low heat and add half as much castor oil as there is herb oil. So if you get four cups of oil out of the herbs, you add two cups of castor oil. Bottle and store.

Cooling Coconut Herb Balm

This balm is beneficial for excess heat, such as when cupping or scraping brings up bright red colors, and for rashes, insect bites, and sunburns. The plantain in the formula is the green leaves that grow all over the world, not the banana relative. Look up pictures of plantain online and try to find which varieties grow in your area; it is quite likely that there is some in your yard! You can also look up Asiatic pennywort to get an idea of what it looks like before heading out to your local Asian food market in search of some. If the Asian food market is Vietnamese, it may be found with the name *pegagan* or *antanan.* It is also known as gotu kola.

All herbs for this formula should be fresh:
- 3 parts plantain
- 3 parts mint

---

60 Castor oil is a purgative and purges the tissue. It pulls from the tissue, including the small blood vessels in the tissue.

- 3 parts coriander leaves
- 3 parts Asiatic pennywort (*bua bok*)
- 1 part kaffir lime leaves
- 1 part lemongrass
- Coconut oil (quantity depends on how much you want to make and the size you choose to make each of the parts)

Chop all herbs as finely as you can. The herbs need to be cooked into the oil using extraordinarily low heat, as this is a cooling balm, and you do not want to infuse it with the qualities of heat. There are three ways to do this:

1. Place the herbs in a glass jar, and cover with coconut oil. The herbs should be packed in tight. Place the jar in a paper bag in the hot sun for about a week.
2. Cook the herbs and oil (herbs packed tight) over *very* low heat for approximately three hours, in a stainless steel or cast iron pan. This method is the most dangerous, as it is very easy to burn the oil.
3. Place the herbs in a glass jar, packed tight. Place the jar in a large pot that is about two-thirds full of hot water. Maintain the water heat by placing the pot on an extremely low-temperature stove top on top of a hot water heater, or in an oven set to about 100 degrees F. Let stand for two days.

When the herbs have cooked into the oil, regardless of method, strain them out. You can use this as is, as a liniment, or turn it into a balm by gently heating it up and adding shaved beeswax. Add some beeswax, let it melt in, then put some of the oil on a spoon and put in in the freezer for a few minutes to solidify. If it is not as firm or thick as you would like, add more beeswax. Continue until you get a balm solidity that you like. While the mixture is still warm, pour into containers of your choice, and let sit until cool and firm.

Healing Salve

This simple, gentle salve is simply amazing. It is excellent on burns, including sunburns and severe burns, and it assists in the rapid healing of traumatic injuries in which the skin and tissue are broken. You will have to find a source of fresh Asiatic pennywort and fresh turmeric. Some Asian food markets carry both.

- 4 cups packed fresh asiatic pennywort
- 4 cups sliced fresh turmeric
- 1 gallon coconut oil
- 2 cups grated beeswax [61]

---

61 Vegans can substitute shea butter for beeswax, although of course it is not Thai. The benefit of beeswax is that it softens the tissue and the skin, helps with adhesions and abnormalities in the skin, and helps to purge toxins. In a healing salve it brings healing properties.

Use scissors to cut the asiatic pennywort into smaller pieces, and gently crush the turmeric in a mortal and pestle. Cook the herbs in the coconut oil over extremely low heat for three to four hours, stirring frequently but not constantly. Make sure the temperature does not get too hot, as if the oil burns the entire batch will have to be discarded. Strain out the herbs, and return the oil to the heat. Add the beeswax and stir until melted. Pour into containers of your choice and allow to sit until cool and firm.

Scar Tissue Poultice

This poultice should be used as part of the scar tissue protocol found in the Physical Therapies chapter.

- 5 parts fresh Asiatic pennywort
- 3 parts fresh turmeric
- 2 parts coconut pulp
- 1 part fresh ginger

Mash all of the herbs in a mortal and pestle, and apply to the area in need. Alternatively, you can use dried powdered herbs and mix them with coconut oil instead of using the coconut pulp, to make a thick paste.

Heating Liniment

This all purpose heating oil can be used to treat scar tissue, and also as after cupping. It is used in the scar tissue protocol in the physical therapies section.

- 2 parts ginger
- 1 part cinnamon
- 2 parts black pepper
- 3 parts safflower
- 2 parts chili pepper
- 2 parts nutmeg
- 2 parts Asiatic pennywort
- Sesame oil
- Castor oil

Fry each herb separately in sesame oil, for ten to fifteen minutes. Strain out the herb, and set the oil aside. Use new oil to fry the next herb. Strain out the herb, and mix the oil with the previous herb's oil. Repeat until all herbs have been cooked and their oils mixed. Add the castor oil, and you are done!

Some Internal Formulas

While people can have allergies to anything, unless otherwise noted, these formulas are gentle herbal remedies that should not cause adverse reactions when interacting with prescription medications. I have tried to choose internal formulas for issues that are common and likely to come into a bodyworker's sphere of community, in the spirit of a Thai medicine practitioner knowing a bit from each root of Thai medicine, even if they do not specialize. For more serious or rare imbalances, you will need to refer your patient to internal medicine specialists, be they in a traditional or a biomedical system.

Seven Peppercorns

It is said that the Buddha himself instructed the forest monks of his time, who had no easy access to medicine, to swallow seven whole peppercorns each day. The seven peppercorns would go a long way toward keeping their bodies healthy, and could be used by all elemental constitutions and balances. Eating seven peppercorns every morning prevents gas, kills bacteria, moves the blood in your body, increases general movement, reduces minor inflammation, and prevents you from getting food poisoning.

Try to find quality peppercorns, that are fat and round and a rich black, perhaps even slightly oily. Swallow them whole like pills, with warm water. I have found that when I follow this protocol, and encourage my family to do the same, we suffer less illness in our household.

Sên Infusion[62]

This infusion, along with the Tissue Softening Infusion in *Thai Herbal Medicine,* is an excellent bodywork assistant, and I recommend that all massage therapists keep some of both on hand. It moves the Wind, making sure that energy is flowing through the *sên,* and helps to gently detox the body. All the herbs are dried, and the parts are by weight. Mybrolan, which can be ordered from Ayurvedic herb suppliers, is astringent, bitter, and sour, so some people will find the taste unpleasant.[63] Add extra honey in the infusion, if this is the case.

- 5 parts Sichuan lovage
- 3 parts clove
- 2 parts fennel
- 1 part black pepper
- 1 part mybrolan (haritaki)
- 1 part cinnamon

---

62 These infusions are what you might think of as teas. Technically, tea is a specific plant, but colloquially it has come to be used for any herbal infusion. Here we will use the more correct term, but the process is the one you are familiar with, of pouring hot water over herbs and letting them steep.

63 The way that we do or do not taste bitter is determined by genetics. Some people don't taste bitter at all, others only mildly, and some very strongly.

Loosely crush the herbs in a mortar and pestle, and use one tablespoon of herbs for a cup of tea. Boil water, and simmer the herbs for about fifteen minutes. It can be drunk with or without honey added to sweeten it. To make a concentrated version, double the herbs, then you can use half a cup of the concentrate and add half a cup of hot water. Concentrate can live for about a week in a refrigerator if you add a little honey or sugar.

Give this tea to patients before massage, and it will help to make the work easier. After massage it helps to reinforce the work, so it can be given both before and after. *Sên* infusion is said to be safe and beneficial for everyone, including pregnant women. This tea can be drunk daily, especially if the patient has a lot of toxins or stagnation in his or her body.

Post Bodywork Detox Infusion

This infusion is beneficial after receiving bodywork, exercising, or other activities that cause detoxification.

All herbs are dried and powdered:
- 2 parts Trikatu (Trikatu is made from equal parts dried and powdered ginger, black pepper, and long pepper)
- 1 part fennel
- 1 part clove
- 1 part nutmeg
- ½ part licorice
- A little raw sugar
- Put a teaspoon of powder in a cup with hot water and sugar to taste.

Pepper Garlic Cardamom Infusion for the Common Cold

This simple tea is excellent for kicking out a cold, if caught early enough. Like all cold formulas, it must be used at the onset of the cold, before the illness has fully lodged itself in the body. Once the cold has truly set in you can still use this to help the body to cope with the illness, but the cold will have to run its course. You could also try the Lime Cold Curing formula in *Thai Herbal Medicine*, another excellent cold formula for colds with sore throats.

The formula given here is better for sniffly, sneezy, feeling-cold colds. The first symptoms of a cold are usually mucous. If the cold turns into a fever, it indicates that the Water element has created a buildup of toxins. Bitter herbs, cupping, and saunas are all recommended.

- 5-7 whole black peppercorns
- 1-3 whole green cardamom pods
- 1 clove garlic
- 1 tablespoon honey
  (local raw honey, if possible)

In a mortal and pestle, grind the peppercorns to a powder. Add the seeds from inside the cardamom pods, discarding the husks. Grind the seeds to a powder with the pepper. Add the garlic and grind until you have a mash. Place the mash in a cup, add the honey, and fill the cup with hot water. Mix and drink.

Tea to Calm the Mind

This is an easy, little, magic solution to calm the mental Winds when someone is experiencing anxiety and mental chaos. It's just jasmine green tea, but the way it is made is important as it flushes out the main caffeine aspect of the green tea and allows the Wind-calming qualities to dominate. Oftentimes, when a friend visits me in distress, I will make a cup of this tea for them without telling them the purpose, and happily watch as they sip the tea and visibly calm. My teacher first recommended it when my son was in the second grade and experiencing some anxious fears. It was lovely to watch the calming effect.

- 1 jasmine green tea bag or tea ball

Pour one cup of boiled water over the tea and steep for thirty seconds. Pour out the water, and pour a second cup of water over the tea. Again allow to steep for only thirty seconds. This time remove the tea bag/ball and drink the tea. Add honey to taste, if you like. This can be drunk before bed and will not cause sleeplessness. Green tea prepared this way is a heart tonic.

Infusion For Malabsorption

This tea is for when you see the scalloped tongue edges that indicate that a person is not properly absorbing the nutrients from the food they are eating.

- 3 parts loosely crushed nutmeg
- 2 parts sliced ginger
- 1 part loosely crushed clove

Use about 1 tablespoon of the herb mix for a cup of tea. Pour boiled water over the herbs, and steep for fifteen minutes. Sweeten with honey, if desired. Alternatively, you can use all dried and powdered herbs, putting about a half teaspoon of the powder mix in a cup with hot water.

Infusion for the Menses

This infusion is primarily for when a woman should be bleeding but is not.

- 3 parts long pepper
- 1 part cinnamon
- 1 part clove
- 2 parts safflower
- 1 part black pepper
- 2 parts calamus

Grind all herbs until they are almost powder. Pour a cup of hot water over approximately one tablespoon of herb mixture, and steep for fifteen minutes.

Blood Formula

Traditional Thai Medicine states that if you can heal the blood, you can heal the entire person. It is also said that whenever you treat someone you must do two things: balance the elements and treat the blood.

There are three aspects of blood that must be addressed. First, the Water aspect, which is the fluidity, viscosity, coagulation factor, and purity of the blood. The Water aspect is cared for by using Sour taste to clean and detoxify it. The second aspect is the Wind, which is the movement, the circulation of the blood. This includes the beating of the heart and the rhythm of the blood being pumped through the body, as well as the smooth flow of the blood. When people talk about Thai massage caring for the *lom*, it is this flow of blood that is often being referred to. The Wind aspect of the blood is supported through hot/pungent taste, as it disperses the blood.

The third aspect of the blood is the Fire aspect. This is the warmth of the blood, the iron in the blood, and the ability of the blood to perform transformation. Bitter is a tonic to the blood, cooling it when overly hot. The blood must be dispersed, tonified, and purified.

This formula is highly prized. It contains only three herbs but maintains health and longevity, as supporting the blood is one of the primary keys to good health. The black pepper nourishes the Wind aspect, the tamarind cleanses the Water aspect, and the gaduchi controls the Fire aspect, keeping the blood cool in relation to the heating qualities of the pepper and tamarind. The three create a perfectly balanced formula.

> *Equal parts ground:*
> - Black pepper
> - *Borapet* [64] บอระเพ็ด
> - Enough tamarind to make a dry paste

Making sure there are no seeds, cook the tamarind in a little boiling water to make a paste. Add the *borapet* and black pepper, and continue to cook until the paste is quite dry, but can be rolled into small pill-sized balls that will hold their shape. Dry the pills in the sun or in a food dehydrator. Alternatively, you can leave the formula as a paste.

DOSAGE: three pills or one teaspoon of paste daily for a month. Some people choose to take this on an ongoing basis for health maintenance.

Maha Pigat Tosa Bencha Khan

This traditional formula is quite similar to a very popular formula called Benjaoon, which is given in *Thai Herbal Medicine*; however, this one is designed to be altered for individual elemental imbalance and relates directly to diagnosis of feces based on color and smell. Each herb in

---

64 *Tinospora cordifolia.* More commonly known through Ayurvedic medicine as Guduchi.

this formula supports a specific element, and the quantities are adjusted depending on the imbalance or season.

This formula works by calling for individual herbs to be included in specific ratios: for example, one herb will have five parts, one will have four parts, one will have three parts, one will have two parts, and one will have one part. When you diagnose what element is primarily out of balance, that element's herb will be the one with five parts. Going down the list of elements above, the next one down from the one with five parts will have four parts. And the next will have three parts. Here is a handy chart to guide you.

Parts	Earth out of Balance	Fire out of Balance	Wind out of Balance	Water out of Balance	Space out of Balance
5 Parts	Long pepper	Plumbago	Sakhan	Piper chaba	Ginger
4 Parts	Plumbago	Sakhan	Piper chaba	Ginger	Long pepper
3 Parts	Sakhan	Piper chaba	Ginger	Long Pepper	Plumbago
2 Parts	Piper chaba	Ginger	Long pepper	Plumbago	Sakhan
1 Part	Ginger	Long pepper	Plumbago	Sakhan	Piper chaba

Once the formula is made, mix one teaspoon of powder with a half cup of warm/hot water. Sweeten with jaggery in the fall and spring (rainy seasons), honey in the winter (cold season), and rock sugar in the summer (hot season).

Here are further details of the herbs, plus substitutions:
EARTH ~ Long pepper (*Dee bplee,* ดีปลี, in Thai)
FIRE ~ Plumbago (*Chitrak/a* in Ayurvedic medicine; *jàyt moon plerng,* เจตมูลเพลิง, in Thai)
WIND ~ *Sakhan* (*Sakhan,* สะค้าน, has no English common name. Piper cubeb, also known as Java pepper, or tailed pepper, can be substituted.)
WATER ~ Piper chaba (known also as wild pepper leaf, *cha phluu,* ช้าพลู, in Thai, wild betel leaf, and *bo la lot* in Vietnamese. Asiatic pennywort may be used as a substitute.)
SPACE ~ Ginger (*khing,* ขิง, in Thai)

Prasagrapao

This traditional formula is beneficial for treating the digestive Winds. It is beneficial for troubles with indigestion, gas, abdominal pain, bloating, and things of this nature.

All parts are dried and powdered and mixed together:
- 2 parts black pepper
- 2 parts ginger
- 2 parts long pepper
  2 parts garlic

- 8 parts licorice
- 8 parts asafoetida
- 1 part black salt
- 20 parts kaffir lime peel
- 47 parts tulsi leaf

DOSAGE: Take half a teaspoon of powder with warm water, as needed. Listen to your body regarding dosing, but approximately three times a day is normal.

Prasaplai

This traditional Thai formula is for blood. It is beneficial for menstrual dysfunction such as irregularities or abnormal discharge, and is a blood purifier. At the time of writing, the primary ingredient, *plai*, is not easily found outside Thailand, but can be ordered online.

All parts are dried and powdered and mixed together:
- 81 parts *plai* (cassumar ginger)
- 1 part camphor
- 8 parts kaffir lime peel
- 8 parts calamus
- 8 parts garlic
- 8 parts shallot
- 8 parts black pepper
- 8 parts long pepper
- 8 parts ginger
- 8 parts turmeric
- 8 parts black cumin
- 8 parts black salt

DOSAGE: Take half a teaspoon of powder with warm water, as needed. Listen to your body regarding dosing, but approximately three times a day is normal.

Indra's Medicine

This is a special traditional formula that is beneficial for almost any troubles with digestion, including food poisoning, nausea, constipation, and stagnation in the digestive tract.

All parts, except the lime, are dried and powdered:
- 5 parts black pepper
- 1 part black aloe vera sap
- 2 parts nutmeg
- 1 part asafoetida
- 1 part camphor
- Fresh lime juice as needed

Mix all the herbs. Add enough lime juice to form a slightly damp paste. Let sit overnight until it forms a dry paste. Form into small pills by rolling in your clean hands, or with a traditional pill gun.

DOSAGE: Take three to five pills a day for three days.

Stomach Ulcer Treatment Pills

Stomach ulcers need to be treated before you can do other work, such as physical therapies.

- Uncooked white rice for rice water
- 1 part organic unripe banana, including the peel,[65] dried and powdered
- 1 part fresh okra steamed, dried, and powdered
- 1 part dried turmeric powder
- 1 part aloe vera powder

The banana and the okra can be dried in the sun or in a food dehydrator and then powdered with a mortar and pestle. Begin by making rice water. This is done by boiling rice in too much water to absorb it all. Once the rice is cooked, the excess water is drained out, cooled, and set aside for making medicine. The rice can be used to make rice soup.

Mix the powders, then add enough rice water to make a paste. Roll the paste into small pills with your hands or using a traditional pill gun, if you have one. This is time-consuming work, so invite a friend over to make it enjoyable. Dry the pills in the sun on a mesh screen (this can take more than one day, depending on the strength of the sun) or in a food dehydrator set at 116° to 118° Fahrenheit, or 46° to 48° Celsius.

DOSAGE: three pills, two or three times per day. Be aware that this medicine is very likely to cause constipation. The person taking it should drink plenty of fluids, including fruit juices, but they still may experience constipation and should be warned.

Kidney Infusion

The kidneys are directly connected to our essence and vitality and are likely to be compromised in those suffering from depression. Nourishing the kidneys is essential to our well-being. This is a gentle kidney-supporting tea made from ingredients common to most kitchens.

- 3 parts green cardamom pods
- 3 parts coriander seeds
- 1 part fennel seed
- 2 sticks lemongrass
- 1 Asiatic pennywort

---

65 Be sure to use organic bananas, as bananas are an incredibly high pesticide fruit, and in using the peel you use the part of the banana to which pesticides are directly applied.

Loosely crush the herbs, and steep one tablespoon of the mixture in hot water for about fifteen minutes. Drink with or without honey. Alternatively, you can powder the herbs and put the mixture in capsules to be taken as medicine.

DOSAGE: one capsule three times a day. This alternative may be good for children, if they don't like the taste of the tea.

Nausea Slices

Soak slices of fresh ginger in raw honey for one to two hours. Eat about three slices. If you make a larger batch of this and soak it for an extended time (honey is a preservative, so it will last), then eat some of the honey as well.

Sore Throat Slices

Soak sliced garlic in honey for one to two hours and eat. If you make a larger batch of this and soak it for an extended time (honey is a preservative, so it will last), then eat some of the honey as well.

Simple Sore Throat Formula

Grind long pepper to a powder. For this purpose, the traditional way of doing it is to take the pepper and rub it against a stone or a rough clay pot. Mix a half teaspoon with lime juice and a bit of sea salt.

Andrographis for Sore Throat

For severe sore throat with inflammation, you can chew on seven fresh *andrographis* leaves with salt. Swallow them, when done chewing. To be prepared, you will need to buy an *andrographis* plant or grow one from seed.

CHAPTER FIVE

Thai Physical Therapies
Gaai-yá-bam-bàt

THAI BODYWORK is an entire branch of Traditional Thai Medicine that consists of a multitude of traditional therapies, ranging from bone setting (indigenous chiropractic) to use of herbal balms, liniments, and hot compresses. In between is a wide range of bodywork techniques, such as Thai deep tissue massage, passive stretching, and work that focuses on freeing pathways of movement in the body, such as in the tendons, muscles, ligaments, and nerves. Thai bodywork can be calming and relaxing, but also holds the potential to be the most physically intensive deep tissue work I know of. It employs esoteric folk healing techniques, such as Thai fire cupping, Thai scraping,[66] and tok *sên*,[67] and sometimes mingles magical remedies with hands-on feats of neuromuscular and myofascial release.

Being a branch of Traditional Thai Medicine, Thai bodywork is steeped in traditional Thai medical theory. Like Rolfing® and other structural integration modalities it can restructure our body alignment, and like Western medical massage it treats chronic pain and goes beyond to treat acute traumatic injury. Unlike most Western modalities, Thai bodywork integrates a deep, spiritual component based on Buddhism as medicine, and the idea that the mental, energetic, emotional, and physical aspects of our being are not separate.

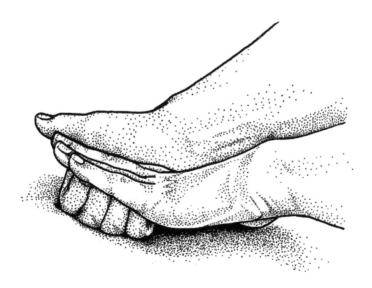

---

66 Use of a tool to scrape the skin (without injuring it), thereby drawing heat and toxins to the surface.

67 Use of a wooden mallet and peg to apply deep percussion therapy.

Until now, Thai bodywork in the West has mostly been enjoyed as a deeply relaxing therapy focused on stretching. This can quite therapeutic, but it is my goal to bring Thai bodywork into an even more therapeutic light. I would like to encourage bodyworkers to learn to do traditional diagnosis and to approach Thai bodywork as a prescriptive physical therapy treatment. This may sound clinical—and to some degree it is—but we must keep in mind what will be learned in more detail in the Buddhism chapter farther along: that Thai medicine insists upon the constant cultivation of kindness and compassion; these qualities are integral to the treatment, but they do not replace knowledge and the application of theory. This is part of what makes it holistic medicine. So whether you choose to employ scraping and deep-tissue techniques, or you choose to give a soothing, relaxing session, the choice should be based on theory and patient need, and be, therefore, prescriptive.

Thai Self-Care
Reu-sĕe dàt dton | ฤษีดัดตน

We start with a brief discussion of *reu-sĕe dàt dton*, the root aspect of all of the externally applied therapies. *Reu-sĕe dàt dton* is the oldest of the medical sciences and is most likely the foundation from which the others grew, as knowledge was first gained through experimentation on the self, then applied to others. Taking care of your own body is vitally important when you care for other people, and understanding as much as possible through direct experience expands a therapist's ability to treat others. This is one of the reasons why oftentimes the best doctors are those who have personally been through suffering and healing.

A *reu-sĕe*, as learned in our chapter on the figureheads of Thai medicine, is a spiritual ascetic/hermit who studies the natural sciences. *Reu-sĕe dàt dton* is the self-care system that is said to have been created by the *reu-sĕe* of long ago. It consists of breathing exercises, self-massage, stretches, chanting, visualization, and meditation. From these exercises come all of the techniques and methods for bodywork, including knowledge of the points, the *sên*, winds, and ways to manipulate the elements in our bodies.

Just as yoga has been diluted from a holistic religious/spiritual path to a stretch class at the gym, *reu-sĕe dàt dton* has, in mainstream Thai culture, been stripped of all of its component parts, except for a simple stretch sequence. These simple sequences are taught at many places around Thailand and can be a good starting place for learning *reu-sĕe dàt dton*, but if you wish to really engage with the practice you will need to seek out a teacher who can instruct in the broader range of the art.

Five-Layer Sequence - Foundation of Bodywork

The most basic Thai bodywork sequence, which can begin and be done anywhere on the body, is to work through the five layers of the body, from superficial to deep. This means that we begin with the skin and work our way through the layers of the body to the level of the bone or the organs, depending on which part of the body you are working on.

Skin

The skin protects us from external pathogens as best it can, but it also protects us from body-work. It may seem subtle and easy to bypass, but the skin layer needs to be addressed before moving on to the fascia and muscles of the tissue layer. One of the best ways to get through the skin layer is to use heating therapies. Always keep in mind with the skin that even as it acts as a protective barrier, it is both an organ of absorption and elimination. We can use the skin to get warmth, herbal remedies, and oils into the body, as well as using it as a doorway from which to draw out toxins, excess heat, and other pathogens.

Tissue

Remember, this is primarily the fat, fascia, and muscle. This level requires more work than the skin level and is where most massage modalities focus. Until the tissue layer has been treated, for the most part you can't go deeper. Access to the tissue layer provides access to the trenches and *sên*, which are mostly located between the tissue and the bone. There are some exceptions, such as the Achilles tendon, where *sên*, or parts of *sên,* are quite superficial, but it's best to stick with the idea of working through the layers in order. In some people, or in some areas of the body the tissue layer will let you go straight to the trenches and the *sên*, but if you haven't addressed the tissue layer then the work you do in the *sên* layer will not be as readily accepted by the body. Have patience. It may take several sessions just to get past the tissue layer in some people.

Sên

Regardless of what else is going on in a session, on some level the *sên* are always accounted for. When we sink our thumbs into the grooves between large muscle groups, we touch the *sên*, giving energy to nerves and veins and arteries, even if we cannot easily distinguish them. At other times, we work directly on the *sên*, plucking at them, rubbing liniments into them, and stretching them. After you have used techniques in an area that release the tissue, always spend some time on the *sên*.

Bone

While external body therapies don't usually work directly on the bones, unless broken bones are being set, the bone layer is addressed through caring for the joints. In many cases, although not all, you can access the joints without having gone through the more superficial layers of the body. It is possible to do traction and range of motion on the joints on many people right away. This is not recommended if you have the time to address the other layers, because when we release the tissue and *sên* layers we often disperse stuck toxins as well as stagnant blood and lymph. These products then have a tendency to get stuck at the joints, which is why you work the joints after the tissue and *sên* layers, even if it is possible to access them immediately.

Organs

Giving attention to the organs is important as they do so much vital work for us, including processing all those toxins that we disperse from stuck areas around the body. Organs are addressed in bodywork both directly through the abdomen, through points that connect to them, and also through caring for the spine, since nerves that connect to the organs must pass through there.

Going through these layers of the body in the proper order applies to just about any therapy in the Thai bodywork tool basket. The generalized sequences that many Thai massage therapists learn have their place and usefulness, but they are not theory, they are not rules, and they are not always applicable. This path through the layers—this is the primary Thai massage sequence; however, listening to the body of the person you are working on is the most important aspect of this work. Depending on what tools are in your tool basket going through the layers can take on hundreds of different looks, but if you slow it down, you will see that someone specializing in scraping, or someone using tok *sên*, or someone doing deep tissue Thai massage, will all, if applying Thai theory, address the layers one by one.

Techniques

Recently a student of mine who comes to Thai bodywork from the acroyoga community told me that some acroyoga instructors have taken to teaching Thai massage with the catchphrase "no extras!" She explained to me that this meant no kneading, gentle strokes, digging around, anything other than the standard compression, line thumbing, and stretching that most people are taught in Thai massage schools.

This idea of "no extras" connects to something I have encountered quite a bit, which is a lack of knowledge about the broad spectrum of possibility that is inherent in Thai bodywork. One of my apprentices confessed not too long ago that she sometimes uses myofascial release techniques while doing Thai massage, even though she "knows it's not Thai," I responded by asking her to break down myofascial release and to please tell me what single part of myofascial release is not found in traditional Thai bodywork, because the truth is, it is all there.

Thai massage suffers from limitations that stem not from the traditions, but from the way it is taught to Westerners. Because of language and time limitations, early on in the developing scene of Westerners coming to Thailand to learn Thai massage, the art was stripped down to a few basic component parts as a way to quickly teach a transient audience. The tendency toward mimicry led each new Thai massage school that opened its doors to Westerners to essentially copy what the other schools were doing, as it was assumed that since it worked at the other school, this must be what people want. Plus it was easily replicated in spas and street massage shops run and worked by Thais who do massage for a living, but have limited healing arts training. And so Thai massage became, to the Western consumer, simply compression, line thumbing, and stretching, often learned in paint-by-numbers sequences. But anyone who has had a number of massages in Thailand will have likely encountered a good deal of "extras" in the work. This is not because therapists are deviating from tradition, but rather because Thai bodywork is a very old healing system that has had a long time to discover a plethora of techniques.

When I rack my mind, in twenty-something years as a massage therapist, there are very few techniques found in Western bodywork modalities that are not found in Thai medicine. Everything that any Rolfer™ has ever done to me, yup, it's here. All those fancy and often branded technique names like petrissage, tapotement, myofascial release, Trager®, effleurage, cross-fiber friction...? It's all here, in truly roots traditional Thai bodywork. They don't use the same names, and they don't always employ the same view of purpose, but the manipulations are the same. This is logical, because if you touch bodies for long enough, in any culture, in any part of the world, you are going to find many of the same truths, for bodies are bodies all over the world.

Of course, traditional Thai bodywork doesn't include every possible therapy. There are things such as the use of essential oils that come to Thailand from the West. And many techniques can be found in Thailand today that are straight up from other Eastern cultures, such as Chinese foot reflexology (in Thailand for about the last 30 years) and Tibetan singing bowls. We live in a very global society right now, and both new and old ideas are constantly being imported/exported all over the world. But when it comes to straightforward manipulations to the physical body, Thailand has a long history of extensive techniques that reaches way beyond compression, thumbing, and stretching; it is inclusive of just about everything I have seen being done in Western body therapies, plus a lot of stuff that isn't being done in the West yet.

During my time living in Thailand, one day I got to sit with my teacher as he translated lists of techniques from various old Thai teaching texts. The following compilation of techniques comes from that day, with techniques unique to northern Thailand, stemming from Lanna culture, added by my teacher. I provide rudimentary instructions for most of the techniques, knowing that people who are already trained in bodywork will immediately understand many but not all of them; for those who have not studied bodywork they may be a little baffling, for bodywork is inherently a physical study that must be learned from a real live teacher.

Techniques Tool Basket

Remember, no matter what technique you are doing, paying attention, listening to the patient's body, being present and in touch, is what makes the work effective, kind, and real.

Pressing/Compression

This is simply applying gentle to deep pressure. Pressing gently primarily affects the skin layer of the body. Deeper compression is used for the tissue, sên and organ layers. To effect changes in these deeper layers, compression should be strong and held steadily for longer periods of time. When I first discovered Thai massage I was, like so many people, enamored with the complicated beautiful stretches. Now it is compression that dominates my work and strikes me as being one of the most therapeutic techniques. It is so simple it can be overlooked, but the power of deep, sustained compression to effect lasting changes on the body is really quite amazing.

Rubbing

Rubbing is the application of vigorous friction with your palms. It affects the skin layer by stimulating the skin, and also through bringing circulation to the surface, causing warmth and distribution of nutrients and oxygen.

Rolling

To roll, place the bone edge of the middle of your forearm on the body, and roll it away from you. Try to use your gentle body weight to push the roll instead of using muscle strength, and make contact with the center of your forearm so that your bone rolls into the tissue. Rolling primarily affects the skin and tissue layers of the body, depending on the depth of the work being done, and it is also used on the organs. Press the tissue as if you are pressing toothpaste out of a tube.

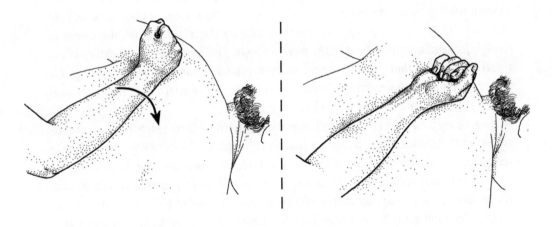

Forearm Roll - start   Forearm Roll - end

Thumb-Pressing Trenches

This is one of the first things taught in most Thai massage classes and is a staple of Thai bodywork. The pad of the thumb is used, not the tip (unless your thumbs simply will not bend), to apply pressure and sink down into the grooves between major structures such as muscles and bones. Be sure to have your body in a position where your thumbs show where the force should be applied, but it is your body weight that delivers that force. Some trenches are very small, in which case fingertips will need to be used, but I shall call it thumb pressing universally, for simplicity. This is not the same as point work, so don't hold thumb presses for an extended period of time in one spot. The overarching reason for thumb pressing is to encourage proper movement, so it is not stationary work. The trenches are thumb-pressed for the following purposes:

TO STIMULATE THE SÊN ~ In this case you are able to sink your thumbs down into the trench, where you will make contact with a multitude of veins, nerves, arteries, tendons, and ligaments. As we know, touch awakens the body and brings body awareness to an area, and with body awareness comes body self-healing and connectiveness. This form of thumb pressing should be done with a straight-down pressure, with thumbs either side by side or one thumb on top of the other. This is done in both directions along the trench, and in most cases which end you start at does not matter.

TO MAKE SPACE ~ The trenches should be places of space, so this work is to free them from obstruction. If you have released the tissue layer but still cannot easily sink your thumbs into the trenches, then your thumb work here is about thumb compressions that create space in order to allow the *sên* in there to breathe, and also so that you will be able to stimulate the *sên* directly. This again uses a straight-down thumb pressure, with one thumb atop the other or both going in simultaneously side by side. This is done in both directions along the trench, and in most cases which end you start at will not matter.

TO MOVE THINGS IN A PARTICULAR DIRECTION ~ Oftentimes, we want to encourage flow of blood, lymph, water, and energy in a particular direction, such as when we want to move toxins away from an injury site, or when we direct flow in a depleted person toward the core (more on all of these choices in the Treatment section below). In this case, you thumb-press in a thumb-over-thumb walk up the trenches. One thumb sinks down into the trench, then as that thumb is being released, the other thumb sinks down a step farther along the path. Think of this as being like squeezing toothpaste through a tube. When doing this kind of work, you choose your direction and work only in that direction.

Heating

Heat can be applied through simple hot packs, hot herbal compresses, and also through the use of herbs with heating qualities that are found in herbal heating balms and liniments. Heating primarily affects the skin and tissue layers of the body. It is extremely effective for relaxing bound-up skin and tissue, increasing localized circulation, relaxing the mind, and cleaning the lymph.

Spreading/Unfolding

This technique uses the palms to sink slightly into the body and glide/push the top layer of skin and tissue. Using both hands, each slightly overlaps the other, one after the other, pushing out in opposite directions. This technique is mostly for relaxation.

Squeezing

Just like it sounds, this involves grasping the tissue and squeezing it. Squeezing can also be done in a wringing out sort of manner or by compression from two sides at once. Squeezing is primarily used on the tissue, *sên*, and organ layers and is good for moving toxins.

Kneading

Western massage therapists will know this as petrissage. This is classic massage in which the tissue is grasped and kneaded and squeezed all at once. Kneading is used on the tissue and organ layers of the body.

Beating

In Thai this is called *dtee* (ตี) and Western massage therapists will know it as tapotement. It uses hands, and sometimes tools, to repeatedly hit the body. Beating is an incredibly therapeutic technique, which, while widely known, is often underutilized. It softens and releases stubborn, bound-up tissue, and it is a dispersing technique that breaks up stagnation and stimulates nerves. Beating must be done for about a minute for it to change the tissue, so have patience and stick around. Beating is another of my personal favorite techniques. Like compression, it is simple and highly effective.

Stretching

This is passive stretching, in which tissue and sên are elongated. To better understand when stretching is called for, it's good to know the difference between tense and tight muscles.

TIGHT MUSCLES exist in a shortened, contracted state. They cannot fully elongate. A person with tight muscles may not be able to do something such as bend over and touch their toes. In this case, stretching is indicated.

TENSE MUSCLES can exist in a body that is very flexible and does not need stretching. In this case, the person might be able to bend over and touch their toes, but if you feel the tissue you find they are holding a lot of tension. In this case, they need to be massaged with techniques such as compression, heating therapies, beating, and so forth. You find this kind of tension in most people, even yoga instructors who are super bendy.

Stretching should be done with specific intention and understanding of what it is accomplishing. Many entry-level Thai massage classes teach highly complicated stretches that affect multiple parts of the body at once. These can be fun and showy, but they do not factor in medicinal therapeutic bodywork. As a rule, doctors in Thailand do not do these complex stretches and acrobatics, as they are unstable and imprecise, and it's important to do precise motions. Of course, those who have learned the acrobatic stretches love them, and with good reason: they are fun and beautiful and can feel quite good. My recommendation is to keep them more in the realm of play than Thai therapeutics.

Ironing

Ironing is when you glide your thumb, fingers, or sometimes palm over the body with strong compression, usually employing a balm or a liniment for lubricant. It reaches the level of the tissue and/or sên, and is also used on the organ layer, depending on the depth of compression and the target focus. Ironing releases tension and moves Wind element.

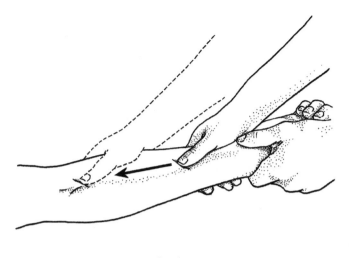

Ironing

Unwinding

Unwinding is done mostly on the limbs. The therapist grasps around the limb with both hands (one from each side) and tugs the tissue first to one side, then to the other. It is a massage technique for the tissue layer that causes release of tension.

Fumbling

When my teacher was translating technique lists from ancient Thai medical texts, he came to this one and said "fumbling." Then he thought about that word and said, "That's really the best translation." Later, he started calling it "fingertip manipulation," which I recognize as being a more respectable term, but I had already grown attached to the word fumbling.

Fumbling is when you use your fingertips to dig in and move tissue around, often in circular patterns but not necessarily. It's one of those techniques (like so many) that most people do instinctively when they massage, even people with no massage training. Fumbling affects the tissue layer.

I have another funny story about fumbling. One day I was with my teacher and a Thai spirit doctor who is one of my teacher's teachers. My teacher was making me demonstrate techniques on the spirit doctor. Now in the US, most people find my bodywork to be extremely deep and intense, but this spirit doctor said (in Thai), "Your fingers are so weak, it is like they are dead."

This rather embarrassing story says a lot about how Thais relate to physical intensity and what is expected in bodywork in different cultures. It is also a good example of what it is like to study Thai healing arts in Thailand—the teachers tend to have a talent for cutting you down to size.

Digging

With digging, you dig your fingertips into the tissue, hook them in, and pull back, pushing and excavating.

Plucking/Strumming

This technique can be quite intense and is used for release and dispersal on the tissue and *sên* levels. It was made popular with Western Thai massage therapists by Mama Lek (a well-loved teacher in northern Thailand, now deceased) and her son Jack Chaiya, who branded it "nerve touch massage." To pluck, or strum, you firmly grasp the tissue or superficial *sên* between your thumb and index finger, with your fingers in a fist fold position. Pull the tissue/*sên* up away from the body, and snap release it.

Plucking invigorates and awakens. It is a forceful stimulating and dispersing technique that can also be used directly on superficial sên. Used on the *sên,* it is beneficial for paralysis, stroke, nerve degeneration, and other instances where the body requires awakening. It also releases stuck tissue, and is the method of manipulation used on the release points found on the Achilles tendon and the sternocleidomastoid muscle. Plucking is similar to scraping, and beneficial for releasing heat. Plucking is a little bit mean, so it is a good idea to let people know that you are aware that it can be uncomfortable. That way they don't think you are accidentally hurting them.

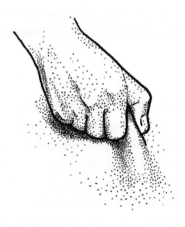

Plucking - start

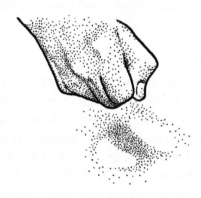

Plucking - finish

Pulling

This is a bit like stretching for the *sên*. It is mostly done on the limbs, where you can put the area, say the forearm, in a lifted elongated position, then stretch it, with a focus on pulling the tendons and ligaments. It should be done slowly, to pull out the Wind.

Scooping

Scooping is basically digging, with a focus on the retractive excavative pulling back. It is done in the trenches and affects the *sên*.

Stripping

Stripping is used on the *sên* and is like ironing, but with the area placed in an elongated position. So, for instance, you can gently stretch out the forearm, then press and glide your thumb down along the tendons.

Twisting

Twisting is exactly what it sounds like. The tissue or the *sên* are twisted to wring them out and stretch them. Twisting is also sometimes used for the level of the bone, such as with spinal twists.

Range of Motion

Range of motion manipulation is for the bone level and is performed at the joints. It is important to know the function of each joint before performing passive range of motion exercises. I mention this because many Thai massage therapists are taught to do circular range of motion on wrists and ankles, when the correct range of motion for both of these joints is flexion and extension.[68] Even if a joint is capable of moving in a different way, with range of motion exercises you want to put the joint through the motions that it is primarily designed for. Only the hip and shoulder joints are designed for full circles.

Range of motion exercises lubricate the joint, remove stuck Wind, and free up the toxins that love to lodge themselves in the joints, causing much joint pain. When you do range of motion exercises on someone, go through each motion nine to twenty-one times. If there is crepitus (nonpainful crackling), continue the motion until the sounds stop.

Vibration

Vibration is another technique that is used for the level of the bone, at the joints. Vibration shakes loose stuck matter and generally loosens the joint. This is generally done after range of motion exercises. Vibration is also used on the organs, helping to disperse toxins. There are three forms of vibration: *jostling*, which is like a quick repetitive bumping or pushing; *shaking*, which is a gentle grasp and shake; and *jackhammer-style vibration*, in which you press your palms down on the area and move them with a very fast up-down vibration. Range of motion exercises and vibration help to get rid of dryness and move Wind. They are not techniques for increasing flexibility.

Traction

The last step in most general bodywork is traction on the joints. To do traction, you pull the limb in a straight line from the joint, opening up the joint and holding for a few moments. This is not about cracking or stretching, although many traction Thai techniques have been misinterpreted as stretches. The goal of traction is to open up the joints, allowing easy Wind element movement for a moment, whereby blood and other fluids that may have become trapped in the joints can flow freely. Always make sure that the joint is in a neutral position.

---

68 Secondarily, inversion/eversion and pronation/supination.

Point Pressing

Thai medicine has multiple point systems: Neuromuscular Release Points, Mental Wind Points, and Wind Gate Points. Here I will explain neuromuscular release points.

Neuromuscular Release Points

These are spots on the body where many sên come together, creating an extra-reactive epicenter for release of tension and invigorated healing. Thai physical therapies tend to be very "on the body." or "what you see is what you get." What I mean by this is that, unlike some systems that use distal referral, the Thai points primarily affect the area directly near them. Distal referral, found in Trigger Point Therapy and traditional Chinese medicine, works on the idea of working on a point in one place on the body in order to affect another place, possibly far away. In Traditional Thai Medicine, if you push on a point near the knee, the knee should be what you are attempting to help. Of course, because the points usually occur where there is a gathering of *sên*, and since *sên* are pathways of movement, it is not uncommon for point work to be felt distally; because this reaction is unreliable, this is seen as more of a side effect in Thai medicine rather than the purpose of the work.

Neuromuscular release points are primarily for treating the tissue layer. Work the point if the area is blocked, bound, or injured, after first addressing the skin and doing at least some compression on the tissue. They can also be worked after the *sên*. Release Points can vary in size. While most will be pressed with the therapist's thumb, some are larger and can take an elbow, and some are tiny, requiring that a small finger.

TO WORK RELEASE POINTS:
1. Press in to one-third of possible depth, with patient inhalation.
2. Hold the point during patient exhalation.
3. On the next inhalation, press in two-thirds of possible depth.
4. Hold with exhalation.
5. On next inhalation, press in to full depth of the point. Hold for a few breaths, and release on an exhalation.

Remember to listen to the body. Step-by-step instructions are a guide, but paying attention to what the body is telling you is ultimately more important. For instance, with the points, if you are present and listening, the body will tell you when you can sink farther in, and when to hold. Hold until you feel the release, then come gently out.

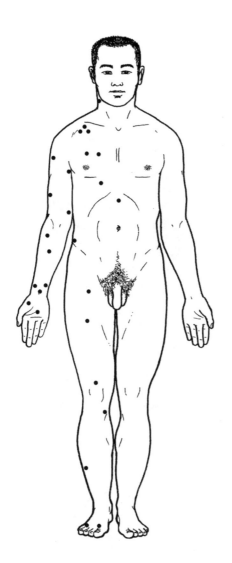

Release Points
Anterior

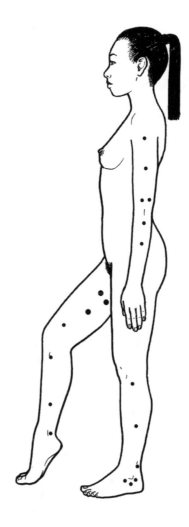

Release Points
Side

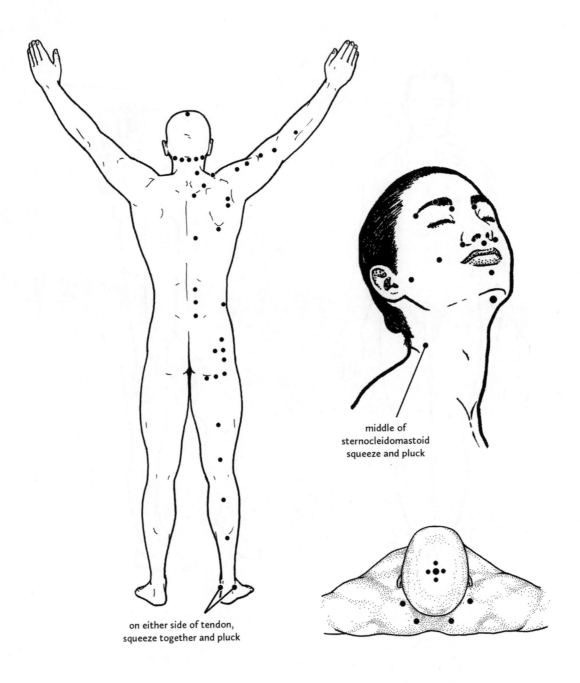

middle of
sternocleidomastoid
squeeze and pluck

on either side of tendon,
squeeze together and pluck

Release Points

Posterior

Release Points

Head and Face

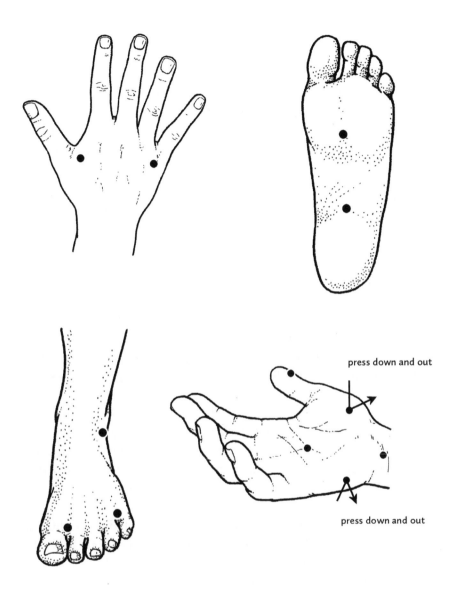

press down and out

press down and out

Release Points of the Hands and Feet

Additional Therapies

In addition to the bodywork techniques listed above, there are many more Thai physical therapies. Most of these require special training that is beyond the scope of this book, as they need to be taught in a live class. But for your edification, I will provide basic information about them here. These therapies are generally used independently or in conjunction with the massage techniques already provided. Most traditional doctors who specialize in bodywork know and use many of these treatment options. I strongly recommend that Thai massage therapists seek out training in Thai cupping, Thai scraping, the therapeutic use of balms and liniments, and the therapeutic use of Thai herbal compresses—and if you can find someone qualified to initiate you, *tok sên*. These therapies can and will change your practice dramatically, and take it to a new level of therapeutic healing.

Thai Fire Cupping

Cupping is a therapy that uses suction to draw unwanted pathogens out of the deeper layers of the body and up to the skin to be eliminated. Most of the time, glass cups that have had a vacuum created in them through the use of fire are applied to the body. The vacuum creates strong suction on the body, effectively pulling up pathogens. Afterwards, the body is often temporarily marked by *lòm bpít*, coloring that varies according to what imbalances are in the body.

Most Westerners, if they know of cupping, know it through traditional Chinese medicine, but forms of cupping can be found in the indigenous medicine practices on every continent on Earth. The oldest known written medical text, the *Egyptian Ebers Papyrus* dated to 1550 BCE, describes bleeding by cupping. Bruce Bentley, an authority on cupping, states:

> *Its appeal probably began as far back as when people sucked at the skin to relieve stings and injuries. Remember as a kid when you jammed your finger in a door and sucked at it to soothe the pain. That's cupping too. It's about the therapeutic action of vacuum. The North and South American natives performed cupping, as well as throughout Africa...*

The basic idea behind cupping is the same in most systems, including Traditional Thai Medicine. Cupping draws out excess Fire, Water, and toxins from the layers of the tissue and the *sên* so that they can be released through the skin. Cupping is both therapeutic and diagnostic, as the colors (or lack of color) that appear on the skin can be used diagnostically to indicate whether further cupping is required and what the followup care should be.

Scraping
gaan krôot | การครูด

Scraping, like cupping, is more commonly known in the West through traditional Chinese medicine and its Chinese name *Gua Sha*, but it is practiced throughout Asia, most commonly in Vietnam, where it is colloquially called "coining." Scraping uses many similar principles to cupping, drawing pathogens to the surface of the body, where the skin can act as an organ of elimination to be rid of them. Scraping employs tools that have a thin but not sharp edge to gently and repetitively rub the body, bringing up *lòm pbìt* like cupping does, but working more on the tissue layer. Scraping is wonderful for releasing tension and excess heat and detoxing the body. It is one of my favorite therapies, and I cannot sing its praises enough. Like cupping it is both therapeutic and diagnostic, as the colors (or lack of color) that appear on the skin can be used diagnostically to indicate if further scraping is needed and what the followup care should be.

Cupping and scraping can both be learned through other medical systems. However, I want to encourage anyone practicing Traditional Thai Medicine to seek out training in therapies that utilize Thai medical theory, if at all possible. While the mechanics of the treatments are similar across medical systems, understanding how they fit within the specific medical modality you practice will broaden the therapeutic value of the work

Bone Setting

jàt grà-dòok | จัดกระดูก

Bone setting can be either medical setting of broken bones, or it can be the application of traction plus high velocity force that we see in Western chiropractics. Unless otherwise noted, I'll be using the term to describe the latter. Bone setting in Thai physical therapies is extensive, and includes many more bone sets than I have seen in the Western chiropractic field. In many Western countries, only those with particular medical licensing are allowed to do bone setting professionally (defined as for any reimbursement, be it monetary or cookies), but with proper training it can be used freely on friends and family.

Bone setting is beyond the scope of this book. I recommend that anyone wanting to incorporate it into their healing arts tool basket be very discriminating in choosing a teacher. Oftentimes, Thai massage classes teach techniques as stretches that were originally meant as bone sets. This has led to some confusion and not a few injuries. Keep in mind that bone sets are high-velocity moves that should not be done without training. Stretches should be slow and engage the tissue. If you are locking joints, it's a bone set move not a stretch. Forced joint cracking is not recommended for most Thai bodywork treatments. Traction, with a slow steady pull on the joint may cause a crack, but this is the Wind element releasing and is not the same as forced cracking.

Burning

Burning is rare these days but can still be found in the deep north of Thailand. It stimulates the points and *sên* at a very deep level. This can be true burning with scarring, or burning of herbs like the use of *moxa*. Burning might be indicated with areas that are severely depleted (such as when you do cupping and the area cupped is very pale). Burning can be done with or without herbs. For instance, in Lanna medicine, the heartwood of pine trees is used for drying wetness, dampness, problems in the tissue, and for getting rid of ghosts.

Bleeding

Blood letting often brings to mind dramatic scenes of medieval medicine drawing large quantities of blood out of patients, thereby unintentionally hastening their death. Rest assured, this is not what is meant by blood letting in Traditional Thai Medicine. Most blood letting that relates to physical therapies is localized blood letting, in which anywhere from a few drops to a few tablespoons of blood are released through the use of tiny punctures and sometimes suction cups. This is done in areas of chronic pain, acute injury, and when indicated by the colors brought forth as a result of cupping and scraping. The blood letting I have seen, and experienced on my own body, was minimally painful, and the blood that came out was clearly stagnant and toxic, being near black in color and far thicker than healthy blood.

Systemic blood letting, with larger quantities of blood released, is done when there is too much systemic heat, such as with fevers and rashes, and is recommended as maintenance at the beginning and middle of the hot season for very fiery people. These days it is simply suggested that those who need to do this donate blood to the Red Cross, as it is safe, effective, and helps others. My husband, who is quite fiery, has donated blood regularly all of his adult life. Until I studied Thai medicine, I did not fully understand why it was that at certain times of year he would announce that he "needed" to give blood, nor did I understand why he felt so much better after doing so when most people just feel depleted.

As you can see, there are many external physical therapies. Remember, all of these therapies are more effective in conjunction with internal medicine, dietary therapies, life style changes, meditation, and so on. To be a well-rounded healing arts practitioner, it is best not to think in terms of bodywork alone but to see the big picture, and to learn as much as possible about how the different therapies support one another.

Physical Therapy Treatments

Thai bodywork is used to:
- Balance the elements
- Realign the physical structures
- Treat the *sên*
- Clean the tissue
- Treat the organs
- Treat injury
- Increase circulation
- Create a state of calm
- Release blockages and stagnation
- Balance and move winds
- Clean lymph
- As a supportive adjunct therapy
- Relieve aches and pains
- Treat paralysis

Another generalized job of Thai bodywork is to work with imbalance that has become substantial and return it to a state of being insubstantial. What I mean by this is that we take that which has solidified (anxiety turned to knots in the shoulder, germs turned to ache, flowing blood into congealed stagnation, and so forth) and use a variety of therapies to melt it, break it down, disperse it, and generally turn it into a state that the body can process and be rid of.

Preparing to do Thai Bodywork

Clothes

The recipient of Thai physical therapies is usually clothed, but because oils, balms, liniments, poultices, and herbal compresses are used extensively in therapeutic Thai bodywork, there needs to be access to the skin. This is accomplished by having the recipient wear very big, loose clothing that is easily reached under or edged up to expose the body. Thai fisherman pants with an oversized loose shirt is the perfect attire.

Mats

Ideally one would have a massage mat that is about two to three inches thick, made from non-toxic, non-petroleum-based[69] materials that come from a renewable resource. The mats we use at the Naga Center are made from natural latex that comes from the sap of rubber trees and has the proteins that cause latex allergies washed out. They are actually manufactured as natural pillow toppers, but we repurposed them in order to meet the comfort, health, and environmental standards that I wasn't finding in other mats being sold to massage therapists. It's lovely to work on high-quality mats, but the truth is that one of the things I love about Thai bodywork is that it doesn't have to be fancy and can be done anywhere. I can do Thai physical therapies on a gym mat, a bed, with the recipient sitting in a chair, really anywhere. So if you don't have the financial means or access to your perfect idea of a massage mat, make do. Use camping pads, blankets, the cushions from outdoor lounge chairs, whatever you have at hand. Make it as fancy or simple as you choose or can. If you do outcall work, I recommend getting an inexpensive tri-fold gym mat with a handle. Gym mats might not be traditional, but they are used all over Thailand; they clean up well and are durable.

Environment

In the West, we like to do massage in a small private room with low lights, candles, silent people, and soft music. And this is lovely. However, like the perfect mat, it's not necessary. Thai healing tends to happen in open rooms with multiple people, laughter, kids, food, phones ringing, and a semi-stray dog wandering about. It's folk medicine. It can happen in a fancy spa or it can happen in a barn. What makes it work isn't the setting; it's the readiness of the patient for healing, and the skill and focus of the practitioner. The more complex the work, the better it is to have a quiet environment for better focus, but it isn't always necessary to create a perfect setting to do healing arts.

Touch

One of the most important lessons that can be learned about touching is this: We can never simply deliver touch; we are always touched back by whatever it is that we make contact with. We are always receiving information in return. If you are new to touching bodies the informa-

---

69 Poly-foam is petroleum based and offgases toxins for a very long time.

tion won't be clear, but as you touch more and more people it will begin to tell an ever more complex story. It's not a story that can be taught in a book like this. It's a story that is learned through your sense of touch alone. I can talk about bound-up tissue, and I can talk about areas that "feel dead," and I can talk about weak tendons, but in truth, the only way to become proficient at finding these places on people is to touch so many people that you know without thinking about it what is healthy and where something is amiss.

Therapist Body Mechanics

Almost everything I say has exceptions. In my classes I will say, "Always have straight arms" and then find that the next move I am showing them requires bent arms. So I approach body mechanics with the thought: *Here is the ideal. Since it won't always be possible, work from the ideal as much as you can. That way, when you have to use your body in a less ideal manner, you'll be able to because you weren't abusing it throughout the whole session.*

For the most part, you want to have straight arms, a straight back, the soles of your bare feet on the floor, and the weight of your body delivering the force. The straight arms are because anytime you have a bend, there is an energetic cutoff. I mean energetic in the metaphysical sense, but I also mean it in a very tangible way. With straight arms, you can sink your body weight into your work, but with bent arms that weight won't go all the way to your hands, and you will have to use muscle strength from the bend down. The soles of the feet on the ground are also about energetic cutoffs, as the soles of our feet are receptive, and it's important to pull up Earth energy into your being as you work.

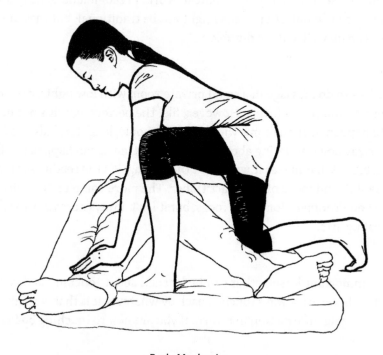

Body Mechanics

Whatever part of you is making contact, be it your hands, your thumbs, your elbows, your knees, or your feet, think of that part as having two jobs: to be a placeholder and a conduit. What I mean by this is that if you are going to do a compression with your palm, you gently place your palm where you want the compression to occur, silently saying to yourself, *Here, here is where it goes.* Then you lean your body into it, bringing the force of the compression from your whole being, through your straight arms, and conducted through your hand, into the patient.

Never use muscle strength if you can use your body weight. When we muscle our way in we must create tension in our own bodies that we then transfer to the patient. If you can sink rather than muscle your way in you can work deeper, being less abrasive. By letting our fingers, thumbs, hands, knees, and elbows simply be placeholders and conduits, we bring our whole body to do the heavy work. Even if the work you are doing is gentle, having the whole of your body behind it keeps it controlled, steady, and grounded.

Focus

Whenever you are doing healing arts work, it is considered best to know what you are doing, be focused, and be deliberate. With Thai bodywork, only work one part of the body at a time. If you have been taught Thai massage sequences that utilize a lot of bilateral work, such as palm-pressing two legs at once, work on becoming accustomed to only doing unilateral work. The reason for this is twofold. One, the body is not a mirror reflection of itself: what is going on on one side of the body is rarely the same on the other side, and so rarely requires the exact same work. And, two, to do truly therapeutic work you must concentrate on what you are doing. If you are pressing two different places, which one are you giving your attention to? Is your mind split between the two? Can you really and truly track the information that the patient's body is giving you in each place and adjust your work accordingly?

Another factor that arises in a lot of Thai bodywork is the tendency to do great big physically intensive complicated stretches that target multiple parts of the body at once. If you do not know what is supposed to be affected by a stretch, it is best to stick with simpler stretches that have a direct focus.

Responsibility

Anytime you do bodywork you take responsibility for someone's physical and emotional safety. For this reason, it is important to only do what you are trained to do[70] and to err on the side of caution. This said, I like to give a lot of responsibility to the person I am working on. This is what I tell people:

> *Thai bodywork can be very gentle, or it can be very physically intense, depending on what is needed and what you are up for. I invite you to notice the difference between pain and injury. Never let me or anyone else injure you, but how much you allow for this treatment*

---

70 Unless you have someone like my husband who agrees, with full understanding of the dangers, to be your guinea pig over and over, despite having once partially dislocated his shoulder while practicing something I shouldn't have been practicing.

to be uncomfortable at times is up to you. It's about your body, not my agenda. If anything I do doesn't feel right or is working at a level that you just aren't up for today, tell me. If you have to pee, if you are cold, if I'm working too deep, if I'm working too soft, if I was working too deep and you told me and now I'm working too soft, or any other thing is going on that you want changed, I expect you to take full responsibility for informing me.

This might seem a bit like overkill, but anyone who has been in the massage business knows that most people will not speak up for their needs while being massaged. So I just like to make sure that the ball is firmly in the patient's court and that they have as much permission as possible to effect a change if needed.

Prayers

I use the word "prayer" without attachment to it being connected to religion or any particular belief. You could change it to "request" or "wish" or "setting intention." Whatever terminology you like, anytime that you do Thai bodywork on someone, the treatment should begin with a moment that is kind of like a mini *wai khru*, in which you silently request guidance and protection in your work, and it should end with a moment in which you wish the person you have been working on well. This ending is like sending the person *metta*.[71] These little silent prayers bookend a Thai healing arts treatment. If you are trained to do more elaborate Thai ceremony in conjunction with healing, then you will also do this, but these more elaborate trainings must be done with a qualified and initiated teacher and cannot be taught in a book if one is following tradition.

Odd and Even Numbers

In most cases, you are not counting the number of times that you do something to the body; however, if for any reason you are counting, bodywork techniques are generally done an odd number of times. The goal of physical therapies is usually to increase movement, freeing up range of motion to joints, muscles, thoughts, and so on. Energetically, odd numbers promote motion, while even numbers promote stability. This is why a four-legged stool is better for standing on than a three-legged stool.

Breath and Bodywork

In the West, most physical therapies, including most massage modalities, advocate that if you are following the breath of the patient, you apply strong pressure or move into deep stretches with the exhalation of the patient. One finds a similar approach with modern yoga, in which we go into the intensity of a stretch with our exhalations.

In Thai medicine the opposite approach is taken. If you are doing Thai self-care exercises (*Reu-sĕe Da Ton*) you inhale, not exhale, with the intensity of a stretch. Likewise, if you are doing something that you know could be particularly intense, painful, or challenging in a bodywork

---

71 Goodwill, or loving kindness

treatment session, you do it while the patient is inhaling. If it is appropriate to be interactive, you can ask the patient to inhale to the challenging spot, bringing breath to it as you work. Conversely, the therapist is usually exhaling as they apply deep pressure. This is because it helps us to not transfer stress into the patient and to continue to send energy as we work. It may be of interest to note that even Indian yoga at one time worked with the breath this way, and that it is only in modern times that the breathing pattern has been reversed.

There are exceptions to this rule, though. If you are working on someone's abdomen, or putting them in a stretch that folds or presses on the abdomen, it may be necessary to have them exhale rather than inhale. I want to note that I do not tailor every move to the patient's breath; to do this would make each treatment session last overly long and is unrealistic. I focus on the breath, as needed, such as when techniques applied are particularly intense or somewhat painful, or when using stretch techniques that clearly benefit from breath involvement.

Treatments

If you have bodywork training, you can take the techniques outlined above, and use them to create bodywork treatments with no further instruction, so long as they made sense to you. Work through the layers, use all techniques at your disposal, stay aware of what part of the body you are on, and why you are doing each thing you do, use the theory you know, and use common sense.

What follows are many different approaches one can take to a bodywork treatment session. Decisions of which protocol to follow should be based on understanding of theory, imbalance causation, elemental states, and the individuality of the person you are working on.

Basics

We'll start with generalized treatment protocols that utilize the techniques outlined above, and are accessible to most who have bodywork experience, and then move on to some more specialized treatments. Unless otherwise noted these are for systemic treatments.

Patient is fatigued, with energy pooling down low

This is often found with people who work manual labor jobs, on their feet all day. Begin at the feet, and work your way up the body toward the head. In this circumstance, the goal is to bring the energy up, taking care of the fatigued and possibly achy feet and legs, then bringing contact to the upper body, finishing there so that the patient is left with a connection to their upper being. Use invigorating techniques like rubbing and beating, and work at a slightly fast pace. Most introductory Thai massage sequences work in this directional (feet up) because they are designed to be generic treatments that will benefit as many people as possible. Thailand, while rapidly modernizing, is still a very agrarian culture, with a majority of people working in agriculture, construction, and other physically demanding jobs that cause this sort of depletion.

Patient is caught up in their head and cannot stop thinking

In this case the patient may be fatigued, but it is due to stress and likely lack of sleep. This is common with those who work mentally challenging jobs, such as those that are computer based, strategic, or otherwise intellectually focused. It is also common with people going through stressful times, such as divorces and other personal life challenges. Care for them by beginning at the head and working down the body to the grounding feet. Use soothing oils, floral scents (they calm mental Winds), work at a steady pace, and avoid complicated positioning.

Patient is bursting with energy, cannot calm, strong energy

This is usually excessive Fire. We will focus on elemental balancing sessions farther down, but for simple directionals, begin at the core and work your way out each of the five limbs,[72] applying traction to the fingers and toes. Think of this as taking that center of excessive energy and dispersing it out the body and finally pulling it out the feet, hands, and the top of the head.

Patient is weak and depleted

Here we are talking about someone who is very depleted. Likely they are pale, lacking in vitality, probably longtime sleep deprivation, stress, or illness. Begin at the extremities, and work in toward the core. Do heating therapies on the abdomen, such as hot herbal compresses or hot packs. Bring it all to center. Work steady.

Patient has weak digestive fire

This will be indicated by scalloped tongue edges, lack of vitality, and food not being properly digested. They require internal herbal medicine as well as dietary and lifestyle changes for full healing, but bodywork can work as a supporting adjunct therapy. Use the same protocol as for the weak and depleted person above. Begin at the ends of the extremities, and work it all in toward the core. Have your agenda be on bringing the energy to the upper digestive system. Do abdominal work, focusing on the stomach and small intestine points, and use heating therapies on the abdomen.

Patient is retaining Water

This is found in overly moist and squishy tissue, Water-based swelling in the extremities, and often in postpartum mothers. Again the protocol is to begin at the ends of the extremities, and work in toward the core; this time with the agenda of pushing the Water into the abdomen, where it can be properly processed by the organs. Use the salt compress formula found in the book *Thai Herbal Medicine: Traditional Recipes for Health and Harmony* (contraindicated with pregnancy). Apply heating balms and liniments to the limbs, always working directionally toward the core.

Patient has an acute injury

Here we are talking about sprains, strains, contusions and other acute injuries. In most cases, the patient will need internal medicine to assist with healing. For general assistance, begin as close to the injury site as possible without risking causing further injury, and work directionally

---

72 In Thai medicine, the head is considered the fifth limb.

away from the injury. Think about encouraging flow of blood and lymph away from the injury site in order to disperse the gathering of toxins that occur at injuries. Thumb-press the trenches using a thumb-over-thumb walking technique, as used anytime you want to move things in a particular direction. Use cooling balms, liniments, and poultices to bring down inflammation. If you can find an Asian trauma liniment, use this. If there is an open wound, do not apply these products on the open wound, just around it. There are healing balms and salves that are made to be applied to open wounds; if you have access to these, use them. If there is no open wound, and you are trained in cupping therapy, do cupping on or near the injury site. Do not ice the injury.

Patient has a chronic ache, pain, trouble spot

In this case, don't worry about whole body systemic work. Just go straight to the injured area. Begin at the epicenter, work through the layers of the body, and follow the pain. I always start by asking the person, "Does it feel fragile and scared of touch, or does it feel like it wants someone to come on in and really work it?" Most people immediately know the answer. If the former, it's probably actually in an acute phase, in which case follow the above protocol. It is a myth that an injury is only acute for the first three days. Old chronic injuries frequently get sent back to being acute as they flare up and re-injure themselves with ease.

But if it is an ache or pain that is ready to be worked out through more intensive physical manipulations, use all techniques at your disposal. If it is bound with adhesions and tension, use beating, compression, heat, warming balms and liniments, stretching (if possible), and any other therapies you are trained in that seem applicable to the situation, such as cupping, scraping, tok *sên*, and so on. The main thing is that if the complaint is a problem area, it's time to break away from sequence work and get spot specific, because until the problem is resolved, the rest of the body will not be able to relax. If the problem area is near or on a limb, after you have thoroughly worked the epicenter and surrounding affected body, then if you have the time, work the entire limb directionally from medial to distal, from close to the trunk, out to the fingers or toes.

Patient has lack of sensation, paralysis, or disconnected "dead" zones

In this case, you need to stimulate and awaken the *sên*. As much as possible, have your focus be on the *sên*, only giving the tissue layer what attention is needed to access the *sên*. Use plucking, digging, and fumbling therapies directly on the *sên* and in the trenches. Also use invigorating rubbing, heating balms and liniments, hot herbal compresses, and, if initiated and trained, *tok sên*. Anytime there is loss of sensation you must be extra careful not to injure, as the patient cannot tell you if you are being too strong.

Patient has a problem area that cannot be worked on directly

In this instance, work the opposite place. For instance, an injury to the pectoral area that is too fragile to be worked on directly will benefit from work in the scapular area of the back that is opposite the trouble spot. This works on the idea that if you have a ball, and you push on one side, it will have a direct effect on the other side. Or, to put it another way, pressing on one side will create a bulge from within on the other side.

Regarding Sequences

Most of the time when anyone who is not studying Thai therapeutics on a medicinal level learns Thai bodywork, they learn a massage sequence that takes them through a series of techniques in a particular order. These sequences vary slightly from school to school, teacher to teacher, but they generally have more in common than not. Most of the sequences begin at the feet and are comprised of compression, stretches, and thumbing the trenches. Bodywork sequences serve a few important roles in Thai healing arts.

Sequences as Teaching Tools

Sequences are not the mainstay of Thai bodywork, yet they are taught to almost all beginning level Thai massage students, and it should be noted that most Westerners who study Thai massage in Thailand will never be seen as anything other than beginners by their Thai teachers (I know, this is rough, but it is true. I've been a massage therapist for about a quarter of a century, but in Thailand I am always a novice). As a result of almost everyone first learning Thai massage in the form of a paint-by-numbers sequence, there is a belief that this is because the sequence is necessary when doing Thai bodywork. What isn't being realized is that the sequence is primarily a teaching tool. To explain this, I like to talk about Taekwando. (Yup, we are jumping ship for a moment here. Bear with me.)

When my son was quite young, he took Taekwando classes at the local community center. Like many martial arts, Taekwando is taught through a series of "katas." A kata looks like a little one-person dance. When my son was a white belt, he learned the white belt kata. It had twenty-one moves, always done in the same order. Then he became a yellow belt and learned another kata, with another set number of sequential moves, another little dance. When you look closely at the dance, though, you realize that it is a series of offensive and defensive fighting moves. Can you imagine if someone who studied Taekwando was to be attacked and instead of fighting back with techniques based on what was coming at them, they started to do their kata? They would not win the fight right? Because the kata was never meant to be Taekwando; it was meant to teach Taekwando.

Thai massage is like this. It is taught in this beautiful sequential dance through the body, but this dance, while it does have healing arts applications, isn't the keystone of Thai bodywork. It is a teaching tool, and while it is useful in certain healing situations outside of learning, when real pain is presenting, simply defaulting to a predetermined set of moves is much like fighting the attackers by doing your kata.

The sequences feel delicious and are used at relaxation spas and street massage shops all over Thailand, but if you wish to move into the deeper healing potential of Thai bodywork, you must lean how to break out of the box, and make choices based not on what comes next in a sequence, but instead on what is going on with the individual you are there to help. My teacher once said:

> It's important to understand the viewpoint and the theory of anything you are doing. In Buddhism, we talk about the importance of intention, but even more important is the viewpoint. Having right view. So if you say I'll just do the sequence and whatever

happens, happens, it's like throwing a knife off of a building and thinking maybe it will kill someone, and maybe it won't.

If you have learned Thai massage sequences, try to look at each part as a lesson. Break it apart, and think about the different techniques in it. Break it down into the techniques list presented here, and try to determine which layer of the body each technique is affecting. Then think about if you can use the same technique on other parts of the body. Because many sequences are designed by people who have not studied Thai medical theory, you will find that they often don't move through the layers of the body in the right order, and that sequences are often taught without understanding that you must complete each layer before moving on, rather than moving on simply because "this is what's next." As we are about to talk about, sequences do have certain therapeutic application, so you will likely want to re-create your sequence work to be in harmony with the theory, and also to better apply to the situations where it is most useful. And of course, add in extras!

Sequence Work for Circulation

Most Thai massage sequences are designed to release blockages in the legs, thereby freeing the Wind element in an area of the body that tends to get bogged down and stuck. Additionally, the sequences are generally set up to move fluids toward the center of the body, bringing blood and lymph into the core, where it can be properly processed. Basic sequence work stimulates vessels and nerves, bringing awakening touch to the entire body.

Sequence Work for Relaxation

One of the primary benefits of sequence work is to provide a full-body relaxation massage session. This is therapeutically prescriptive in cases of great stress, emotional trauma, sleeplessness, and mental chaos. When doing sequence work for the purpose of relaxation, it is beneficial to incorporate hot herbal compresses and oils infused with floral aromatics, such as jasmine and rose, as these scents calm the mental Winds.

Sequence Work for Calming the Winds

Sequence work is prescriptive for those with agitated Wind element, which is calmed by rhythmic, balanced bodywork. Make sure that in this case you do not increase the Wind element by engaging in lots of stretches, or moving the person around too much. Try to switch sides often enough to avoid imbalance, yet not so often as to be chaotic. See below for more details on calming the Wind element with bodywork.

Bodywork to Balance The Elements

If you take time to consider the experience, qualities and function of the elements, then much of what is needed to care for them, be it nourishing or calming, will be logical and clear. If you can identify which elemental qualities are at play, you can make informed decisions about treatment. For example, if you have a Wind condition that is rough, light, and dry, then you treat it with oil, because oil is smooth, heavy, and unctuous. But if the Wind condition is just too cool, then you could use any warming therapies. Following are some basic protocols for elemental imbalances; however, the more you understand the basic information about the element, the more you will be able to suss out what needs doing on your own.

> *Calming/subduing therapies are to tame an element that is agitated, or perhaps deranged. Nourishing therapies will build or strengthen an element that is weakened or depleted.*

Wind - Calming/Subduing

If you are not doing a spot-specific treatment, do slow rhythmic and balanced or sequential massage, being sure of symmetry. Change sides fairly frequently, so that one side does not get very off balance from the other, but not so frequently as to cause a feeling of chaos. Use oil—sesame oil, olive oil, mustard seed oil, or safflower oil are all good (coconut is too cooling). Do not do a lot of stretching or other techniques that unbalance or move the body around a lot. Do more point work, *sen* line work, and deep compression. Traction will help to create space in the joints. Use hot liniments and balms. Blood stops are also good, as are wet, hot compresses. Unless otherwise indicated, work in both directions.

Do not move your client around too much—think of keeping them connected to the earth. *Lom* can refer to the Wind element in the body, encompassing electrical energy, nervous system, all movement, mental Winds, and breath; it can also refer to spirits and problems that spirits cause for people. Anything that treats the Wind element is going to treat all of these interpretations, so if you don't know the specific Wind that is a problem, use general Wind element calming therapies.

- Slow, rhythmic, balanced
- Same thing on each side of the body
- Oil—sesame, olive, mustard seed, safflower
- Point work, *sên* line work, deep compression
- Not too much stretching or moving
- Use hot liniments and balms
- Blood stops
- Wet, hot compresses

To Nourish Wind

To nourish the Wind element, do a lot of range of motion. Focus on invigorating therapies, and work at a faster pace.

Fire - Calming/Subduing

Do deep work and point work. You can do some stretching, holding the stretches for longer periods of time. You can also combine stretching with point work—working the points while in a stretch. Oil is not usually called for with fire, but if you are going to use oil use coconut oil, as it is more cooling than other oils. Floral waters such as rose water can be a substitute for oil, and are better for fire. Use cool compresses—compresses that contain cooling herbs, such as plantain, roots, Asiatic pennywort, shredded coconut, dandelion greens, spinach, clay, or rice. Rice and clay are both cooling and draw out toxic heat. You can put the compress in the sun or steam it, but do not use while it is too hot. You can also soak the compress in cool water.

Give a smooth and calm massage, but do not work too slowly, as fiery people can become impatient with slow work. Do scraping to release excess heat. Work from the center toward the extremities to disperse heat. Fiery people can usually take (and prefer) deep physically intensive work—and they will not need as much time to process the work as others.

- Deep work
- Point work
- Slow long stretches (not required, but if you are stretching)
- Cooling balms, compresses, poultices, waters, and liniments
- Do specific work

Fire - Nourishing or Building

To nourish the Fire element, do a lot of abdominal work, and when working the extremities, work toward the core. Use warming balms, liniments, and compresses. Invigorate, heat, and enliven.

Water - Calming/Subduing

Do lots of stretching, squeezing, pressing, and twisting (think of wringing out the water). *Sên* lines can be worked, but generally you must be a bit more gentle as watery people injure/bruise easily. Usually point work is not indicated with watery people. Use heating and dispersing balms, liniments, and compresses. A faster pace is helpful with water, as water tends toward being overly sedate. Cupping helps to remove stagnation and toxins. Use techniques that are active to generate Fire element and energy, with a lot of movement. Work toward the center.

- Stretching
- Twisting
- *Sen* lines gently
- Less point work
- Heating and dispersing herbs
- Fast pace
- Cupping

Water - Nourishing or Building

To nourish water, do a lot of stretching and apply oils. Use warm, wet compresses and work slowly.

Earth

Work the feet, and do all the therapies that calm the Water element. While we don't generally tailor a bodywork session for Earth element, it is good to keep in mind that all physical therapies are working on and benefiting Earth.

Treating the Sên

The *sên* are considered and addressed in just about every Thai bodywork treatment; however, if you wish to do focused work for the *sên*, this is quite specific. The purpose is to maintain general health and smooth flow of the pathways of movement. You must still make sure that the skin and tissue layers are letting you in, of course; from there, you employ techniques that treat *sên,* such as ironing, stripping, plucking, certain stretches, and, if you have been trained and initiated, *tok sên.* Here is a general sequence for treating the *sên* through the trenches. In preparation for this work, mix some warming balm with sesame oil. If it is cold, you can mix it with warming liniment, and if it is very hot, you can mix it with coconut oil.

General Sên Oil Treatment

1. Warm up the body, rubbing down through cloth—unless they are cold, in which case, you can use oil.
2. Palm-press (compression) the area.
3. Rub the oil balm mix vigorously into the trench.
4. Slide your thumbs down the trench in one direction, twenty-one times.
5. Make a fist and slide knuckles (other hand cupped, supporting) down the trench seven times.
6. Thumb-press the trench three times.
7. Slide thumbs down a few more times.
8. Slide palms away from you, overlapping one another, down the area.

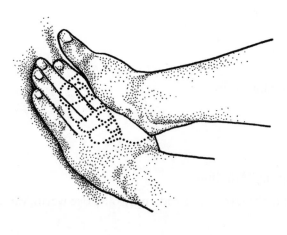

Subtle Wind Gate
(Bprà-dtoo lom) Treatments

It is generally a good idea to work on wind gate points after clearing the skin, tissue, and channels; however, there are times when they must be worked first, such as with patients who have so much pain that they cannot otherwise be touched, or in cases of extreme excess. This method of working with the wind gates is much gentler work than the arterial occlusion popularly known by the misnomer "blood stops." With the more subtle Wind Gate work, the idea is to gently engage the pulse, bringing the body's awareness to its own rhythms and qualities. The therapist isn't so much fixing as he or she is pointing out the problem to the body so that it can adjust itself. Working with the Wind Gates is good for balancing the Winds, high blood pressure, clearing the body, and balancing the flow of movement above and below the Wind Gate.

How to Work the Wind Gates

1. Press in until you feel the pulse. Engage the pulse a little bit, but do not try to occlude it. If it was a tube, it would be pressed down about one-third of the way. Be very gentle and slow and focused. Do not work on Wind Gates in a chaotic environment, or with music playing. You need to be able to tune into the patient's pulses, which is difficult to do with too much external stimuli or the beat of music replacing the beat of the pulse in your awareness.
2. Tune in to the rhythm of the pulse. Listen attentively to it. Try to get a sense of the rhythm and qualities of the pulse.
3. Hold until you feel a change in the pulse—it will speed up, slow down, soften, and so on. Just notice it, don't release.
4. Keep holding until the pulse settles again. This is a like a second, more subtle change, almost like the pulse is settling into the first change. Feeling for it is a bit like looking for something with your peripheral vision.
5. Slowly release the pulse.

   • *In cases of excess*, work the wind gate points first, then clear the channels
   • *In cases of depletion*, clear the channels, then work the wind gates
   • *When you work a wind gate*, you should always feel a pulse and you should never move around

Wind Gate Cautions
   • Use care when pressing on the abdominal (navel) Wind Gate on very thin patients, as it can be pressed into the spine.
   • Wind gates should not be pressed more than three times consecutively.
   • Do not perform Wind Gate compression bilaterally (holding two Wind Gates at once) as this divides your focus.
   • Once you have engaged the pulse, do not move around or reposition in any way.

General Pattern for Wind Gate Work

Generally start with the abdominal gate and work from there. If you are working on the legs just work the legs, beginning with the navel, but don't worry about the arms. When working the Navel Wind Gate, be extra careful with very thin people, as you can compress the descending aorta into the spine.

- **If needing to build strength, energy**, and so on, work toward the abdomen.
- **If needing to balance or disperse**, work from the abdomen toward the extremities.

1. Rub the area being worked (so, if starting with legs, rub the whole leg).
2. Palm-press the area being worked (that is, the whole leg).
3. Do range of motion on the area to be worked (just near the first Wind Gate. So if working the leg, do range of motion exercises on the ankle at this point, then work the Wind Gate, then do range of motion on the knee).
4. Shake the area being worked.
5 Work the Wind Gate as outlined above.
6. Move to the next section of the body.

Wind Gate Protocol for Problems with Mental Wind

Do the general pattern for Wind Gate work, beginning with the neck and moving down the body and out the extremities to the hands and feet. Abdomen can be done after arms, or last of all.

Wind Gate Protocol for Exhaustion and Depletion

Work the Wind Gate points in a star pattern as follows:
1. Work one leg, from foot to hip.
2. Work the opposite arm, from hand to shoulder (so if you began with the left leg, you would now move to the right arm).
3. Work the other arm, from hand to shoulder.
4. Work the leg that has not yet been worked, from foot to hip.
5. Work the abdomen.
6. Work the neck and head.

Wind Gate Protocol for Abdominal Wind

Beginning with the stomach, work out to the extremities:
1. Work the stomach.
2. Work one leg, from hip down to foot.
3. Work the other leg, from hip down to foot.
4. Work one arm, from shoulder to hand.
5. Work the other arm from shoulder to hand.
6. Work the neck/head.

Fingers and Toes

The Wind Gates in the fingers and toes are assisted when you traction them in a long, not jerky, prolonged kind of pull. If you have an accumulation of Wind element in the upper arm, you can move it down, down, down and then pull it out the fingers. It will pop, but this is not a bone-setting crack.

Thai Abdominal Massage / Treating the Organs

Treating the abdomen is of great importance for general health, as this is where our organs are located, which do most of the vital life work. On an energetic level, the abdomen is the seat of vitality, and the source for many basic life forces within us. Unless you are just doing spot specific work on a problem area, and that is all you have time for, every treatment will ideally involve abdominal work. In particular, abdominal massage is beneficial for:

- Low digestive fire
- Treating the organs
- General weakness
- Dispersing Wind element in the abdomen (bloating, excessive gas and belching, and so on)
- Posterior/back issues
- Menstrual cramps
- Constipation
- Removing toxins

There are complete systems for treating the abdomen, but for general massage on the abdomen, simply make sure that you go through the layers of body, just like you would anywhere else, treating organ points, as needed, at the end.

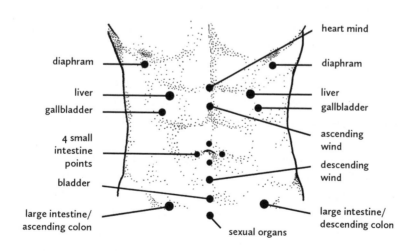

This can be harder on the abdomen, as knowing when you are on the tissue layer, when you are the *sên* layer, and when you are on the organ layer takes time and experience. Techniques such as palm pressing, using hot herbal compresses, thumbing trenches, and vibration are all good for general abdominal massage.

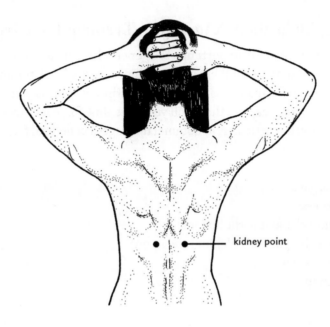

kidney point

Organ Points

Prenatal Thai Bodywork

Prenatal Thai bodywork is nearly entirely done using hot herbal compresses and oils. Standard sequential Thai massage should never be done on pregnant women for two primary reasons: It causes significant detoxification (and detoxing while pregnant can be dangerous), and the stretches often found in standard Thai massage sequences are potentially dangerous due to the presence of relaxin, a hormone that causes pregnant women's tendons and ligaments to loosen. Because of relaxin, it is easy to accidentally overstretch a pregnant woman and cause injury. Do not do thumb pressing of the trenches, deep tissue work or strong stretches, and avoid heating and expelling herbs, including Thai warming balms and liniments, as well as classic herbal compresses.

Systemic or spot specific use of hot herbal compresses makes up the bulk of prenatal Thai massage work. You will have to make your own compresses, as the generic ones that come premade have many ingredients that are contraindicated with pregnancy, including *plai*, an herb found in almost all generic compresses, which is wonderful for the tissue but moves blood too much for prenatal work. Use the prenatal compress formulas found in the Herbalism section on page 140. It is also okay to do gentle point work, gentle palm compressions, and to massage oils into the pregnant woman's skin.

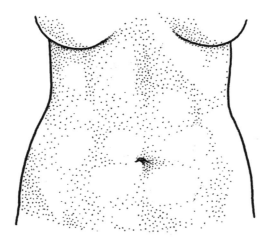

Pregnant women should be worked primarily in the sidelying[73] position, with two pillows under the upper leg, a pillow under the head, and another pillow in front of their body, with their upper arm draped over it. If they need to be placed in supine position, check in first to make certain that they are comfortable lying face up. Toward the end of pregnancy, many women are only able to remain on their backs for short amounts of time before pressure on the inferior vena cava causes discomfort, nausea, and head pain. To avoid this, place them in a recumbent supine position, with pillows under the upper back and head such that they are partially seated. Pregnant women can also be in full seated position, although this tends to be less relaxing. Pregnant women are generally only worked on for about an hour. This is to avoid overworking their body, but also because pregnant women need to eat, drink, and urinate frequently.

Contraindications

- *Do not do thumb pressing in the trenches*, due to detoxification effects.
- *Only perform exceedingly gentle stretches*, if any, due to relaxin.
- *No heating or expelling herbs*, due to the energetics of expulsion.
- *No Wind Gate work (no blood stops)*, due to potential for deep vein thrombosis and many other reasons.
- *No strong compression on abdomen*, due to discomfort to the mother and baby.
- *No deep work on the inner thighs* due to increased blood clotting factors and subsequent increased chance of deep vein thrombosis
- No *plai* or salt compresses, due to drying and Wind-moving potentials.
- *Traditionally bodywork is contraindicated during the first trimester*, when the baby's kwǎn has not yet settled in its body and potential for miscarriage is stronger.

---

73 Lateral recumbent

- Do not use modern massage tables or bolsters that are designed to allow pregnant women to lie prone. While being face down is very appealing to many pregnant women, these contraptions put undo stress on the uterine tendons and ligaments as they are tugged by the pregnant stomach being weighted straight down. Even the ones with straps and such underneath the belly are contraindicated.

Postpartum Thai Bodywork

Traditionally, postpartum women in Thailand spend five days to over a month in confinement, lying by a hot fire, drinking herbal teas, and bathing in herbal waters, with only close family and their midwife around. This time is called *yòo fai* (อยู่ไฟ). They also do herbal women's steams to clean out the vaginal canal and uterus, and eat grilled sticky rice with salt to help dry the uterus out.

In the US, I have observed that the vast majority of mothers I know suffer from varying degrees of chronic illness after they have children. I know several women with endocrine system troubles that keep them sick more often than they are well, and I suspect that traditions such as *yòo fai*, which are found in most traditional cultures around the world, help to prevent this sort of ongoing ill health. All of the traditions that I know of, like the Thai one, acknowledge the depleting quality of pregnancy and childbirth, and encourage the mother to stay very warm and to be nourished with warm teas and foods and to get as much rest as possible. This time also provides a quiet time for the newborn baby to adjust to life outside the womb.

For bodywork, most of the same rules apply to postpartum women as pregnant women, as they generally still cannot lie on their stomachs, and relaxin remains in the body for up to six months. However, at this time, heating and expelling herbs are okay, and even recommended. Classic Thai herbal compresses can be employed, deeper bodywork performed, and heating balms and liniments used (but keep them away from areas where the baby will be making contact with the mother).

Traditionally, a warm clay pot with heated rock salt in it was placed over a towel on the mother's stomach to help reduce excess Water element, and to encourage the uterus to contract to pre-pregnancy size. A salt-drying compress made from rock salt and a small amount of nutmeg and long pepper can be used on anywhere that has excess Water element being retained, including over the lower abdomen to help dry out the uterus (note: this is contraindicated during pregnancy). Postpartum women are encouraged to stay very warm for the first month, and to take herbal steams and saunas frequently.

In the West, a great deal of care is generally given to pregnant women. They are given gift certificates for massage, encouraged to relax, and be pampered. This is all lovely, but I have found that postpartum women have an even greater need for care than pregnant women. Postpartum mothers generally have all sorts of aches and pains, are seriously depleted, and fatigued. They have terribly bound-up tissue in their shoulders and necks from the positions they maintain while feeding their babies, and their forearms tend to be quite bound up from holding babies on hips (this is found in fathers, as well).

Because of how busy they tend to be (no *yòo fai* in the West; it's get back to work, take care of business!), it can be difficult to get postpartum moms to receive care. I stopped doing outcall work long ago, but have maintained an exception for new mothers (as well as people fresh out of surgery), and I always make clear that I can work on them even with baby on the breast or in the arms—anything to make it more possible for parents to get some much-needed care.

Massage to Nourish Essence

There isn't one single treatment protocol for nourishing depleted essence, so you can follow these tips to create your own.

- Do oil massage with raw sesame oil.
- Work from the extremities toward the core.
- Use heating therapies on the core and kidneys, such as hot herbal compresses.
- Do the star gate pattern Wind Gate work.
- Use compresses, oils, candles, and such with good floral smells if you can, including jasmine and rose to calm the mind.
- Do nurturing, nourishing massage, with nothing chaotic or depleting, such as big stretches or strong cupping.

Treatment for Scar Tissue

Warm up the area with massage, then apply the Scar Tissue Poultice on page 144. Leave on for fifteen minutes. Remove the poultice, and do sliding cup therapy if you are trained in this technique. If the scar is near a joint, do a huge amount of range of motion exercises. Put the poultice back on for fifteen to thirty minutes. Remove, and massage a heating liniment into the area.

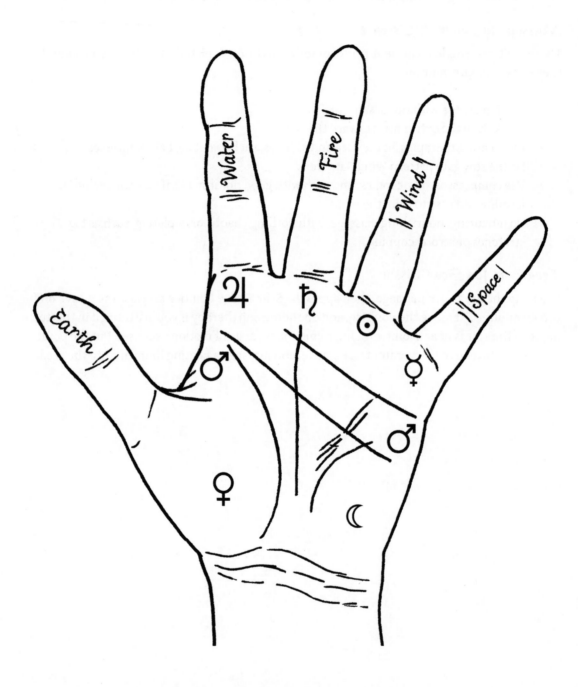

CHAPTER SIX

Divinatory Sciences

Hŏh raa sàat | โหราศาสตร์

THE NEXT ROOT OF THAI MEDICINE that we will discuss is *Hŏh raa sàat*, the divinatory sciences. By this, I mean things such as astrology, numerology, palmistry, geomancy, and many more esoteric systems of divination. In the West, we tend to use these systems to discern probabilities surrounding love, character, and finances. Of course, in Thailand, they do this as well, as people all over the world are interested in these things, but the reason that you find the oracular arts listed as a root of medicine is because in Thailand they use these skills to understand health, disease predisposition, remedial prescriptions, and elemental balance. I have seen various healing arts practitioners, from bodyworkers to medicine men, turn to divinatory arts for extra guidance in determining what is amiss with a patient. Those who specialize in in divination are called *mŏr doo* (หมอดู), which translates as "seer doctor."

Divinatory arts are a mixture of a tool (the divinatory system, such as astrology or tarot) and intuition. It is my belief that the systems are gateways to the intuition. At first, people studying a system of divination will have only the system, and the results will be mixed. But for those who develop a strong sense of intuition and who communicate well with their patients, the results can be startlingly accurate. It is important, though, to avoid the temptation to treat these things as parlor tricks. The seers I have met who have reduced my skepticism have felt free to ask me questions, letting a combination of information from me, information from my palm or the stars or the cards, and intuition come together to form a full and useful picture. They did not feel that they had to prove a magical ability by knowing all about me before I'd said a word.

Thai Astrology - Hŏh raa sàat

You will notice that the Thai word for astrology is the same as the word for this whole root of Thai medicine. This shows the importance of this particular art in the oracular field. The form of astrology used in Thailand is Indian Jyotish astrology, or sidereal astrology. In the West, the primary system used is equinoxal, although sidereal astrology can be found in the West as well. They are quite similar; in fact, equinoxal astrology grew out of Jyotish astrology, which contains all of the familiar planets, zodiac signs, and, of importance to healing arts practitioners, elemental associations. Anyone who has ever said "I'm Aries, I'm a Fire sign," knows on some level that astrology places importance on the elements. While the art of astrology is too vast for this book (and my own knowledge not vast enough), if you choose to study astrology you can combine your knowledge of elements that you have gained here with the study of astrology to form a more complete Thai diagnostic picture. If you add to this the Thai focus on the day of the week you are born on, and an understanding of Thai auspicious and inauspicious days, then you have properly "Thai-ified" your astrological talents.

Day of Birth	Auspicious Color	Inauspicious Color	Deity	Planet	Gemstone
Sunday *wan aa-tít*	Red	Blue	Surya	Sun	Ruby
Monday *wan jan*	Yellow	Red	Chandra	Moon	Diamond
Tuesday *wan ang-kaan*	Pink	Yellow or white	Mangala	Mars	Black sapphire and garnet
Wednesday Day *wan pút*	Green	Pink	Buddha	Mercury	Emerald
Wednesday evening	Grey	Orange or red	Buddha	Rahu	Lapis lazuli
Thursday *wan pá-réu-hàt*	Orange	Purple	Brihaspati	Jupiter	Topaz
Saturday *wan săo*	Light Blue	Black or dark blue	Shukra	Venus	Blue sapphire

Thai astrology has the following elemental associations:

EARTH: Taurus, Virgo, and Capricorn. Planet: Moon and Jupiter
WATER: Cancer, Scorpio, and Pisces. Planets: Mercury and Venus
FIRE: Aries, Leo, and Sagittarius. Planets: Sun and Saturn
WIND: Gemini, Libra, and Aquarius. Planets: Mars and Rāhū

One thing to keep in mind is that elemental constitution is determined at the time of conception based on seasonal, astrological, and genetic factors. However, within the first handful of years of life it is possible, albeit rare, to change the core elemental constitution. This can be seen when an astrological chart doesn't elementally match with an otherwise determined core elemental diagnosis.

Birth Days

An aspect of Thai astrology that is uniquely Thai is the importance placed on the day of the week that you are born on. In Thailand, everyone knows what day they were born, and they find it strange that Westerners usually do not have this knowledge. The first time a Thai monk asked me which day I was born on (in preparation for telling me when I should next travel), he was clearly baffled by the fact that I didn't have an answer. I think that for a moment there he wondered if I might be lacking in some vital mental capacities. Not knowing if you were born on say, a Saturday, is like not knowing who your country's prime minister is (or president, queen, czar, and so on). The day of the week that you were born on determines what color is lucky for you, what color is not, what planet you are ruled by, and what deity you are associated with (and might want to nourish a relationship with). Like an astrological sign, it tells about your character, interpersonal relationships, and financial possibilities.

If you were born on...	Don't do anything auspicious on...
Sunday	Friday
Monday	Sunday
Tuesday	Monday
Wednesday	Tuesday
Thursday	Saturday
Friday	Wednesday
Saturday	Wednesday in the night

Buddha Postures

The day of the week you are born on also connects you to a particular image of the Buddha. Statues around Thailand will frequently depict the Buddha in a variety of eight postures. Each posture is associated with an event in the Buddha's life, as well as a day of the week. So, for instance, I was born on a Monday, and the Buddha image for Monday is the Buddha standing, with one or both hands forward in a gesture of pacification. In Thailand, it would be expected that I would gravitate toward this image of the Buddha, giving offerings and donations to shrines that depict him thus.

Sunday's Buddha Posture

This shows the Buddha standing, with hands folded in front of him. It represents the time just after his enlightenment when he stood and contemplated human suffering, while gazing upon the Bodhi tree that sheltered him during his enlightenment. This image is reflective of kindness, thoughtfulness, and open eyes. It is known as "The Buddha in Pensive Thought" or "The Buddha with Dedicated Eyes" *Prá bpaang tà-wăai nêt* (พระปางถวายเนตร).

Monday's Buddha Posture

This shows the Buddha standing with one or both of his hands held out in front of him, palm/s facing outward. This pose is reflective of a time when he calmed a dispute between relatives. It represents pacification and peace, and is sometimes known as "The Buddha Preventing Calamities" or "The Buddha Making Peace" *Prá bpaang hâam yâat* (พระปางห้ามญาติ).

Tuesday's Buddha Posture

This shows the reclining Buddha on the day of his death. This is not seen as a negative, but brings to mind his final words: "As a flame blown out by the wind goes to rest and cannot be defined, so the wise man freed from individuality goes to rest and cannot be defined. Gone beyond all images, gone beyond the power of words." This Buddha image is called "The Buddha Reaching Nirvana" *prá bpaang săi-yâat* (พระปางไสยาสน์).

Wednesday's Buddha Posture (Day)

This shows the Buddha standing holding an alms bowl. This image refers to a tale of a time when the Buddha visited his father, and his father was saddened to see his son begging; but the Buddha explained to his father the importance of a monk's *pindabat* (alms rounds), how availing themselves to the generosity of others is a service to those who give. This image is reflective of receiving. Wednesday is unique in that it is broken into two sections, with a different Buddha image for those born in the evening. This Buddha is called "The Buddha with Alms Bowl" *Prá bpaang ôom bàat* (พระปางอุ้มบาตร).

Wednesday's Buddha Posture (Evening)

This shows the Buddha sitting in meditation, generally with the attendance of a monkey and an elephant. It is reflective of the Buddha's respect for all living beings, as well as all living beings' respect for the Buddha. This image is called "The Forest Buddha" *Prá bpaang bpàa lay-lai* (พระปางป่าเลไลย์).

Thursday's Buddha Posture

This shows the Buddha in peaceful meditation. It is a simple pose, without story, reminding us of perfect mindfulness. This image is called "The Meditating Buddha" *prá bpaang dtràt róo rěu bpaang sà-màat* (พระปางตรัสรู้หรือปางสมาธิ).

Friday's Buddha Posture

This image shows the Buddha again standing by the Bodhi tree, this time with his arms crossed over his chest. He is recently enlightened, contemplating how to teach the dharma to others. This pose reflects spiritual transformation, as well as the Buddha's compassion for all beings, as is shown by his teaching what he thought to be impossible to teach. This image is called "The Contemplating Buddha" *prá bpaang ram peung* (พระปางรำพึง).

Saturday's Buddha Posture

This image shows the Buddha sitting in calm meditation while a storm rages around him. He is protected from the storm by Muchalinda, the five-headed *naga*. This pose reflects calm in the storm, and in the protection offered by the naga, again we see the respect of all beings for The Buddha. This image is called "The Buddha Protected by the Naga King" *prá bpaang nâak bpròk* (พระปางนาคปรก).

Auspicious Days

Auspicious activities include blessing a new house, getting married, adopting a child, setting forth on a journey, starting a business, and so forth.

Palmistry
Sàat hàeng gaan doo laai meu | ศาสตร์แห่งการดูลายมือ

As with astrology, palmistry—the art of looking at the hands for information about a person's life—is said to come from ancient India. It has spread around the world and is practiced throughout the East and West alike, with some variance but much similarity. In addition to what is seen in the lines of the hand, palmistry looks to the mounts (fleshy mounds) of the palms and the fingers for planetary and elemental associations. In this aspect it strongly resembles, and is a cousin to, astrology. In the marvelous Vedic palmistry book *Introduction to Hast Jyotish: Ancient Eastern System of Palmistry*, the author, Ghanshyam Singh Birla, says:

> *Each element corresponds to a mount and finger that, in turn, correlates to one of our physical senses. The formation of our mounts and the fingers determines to what extent we have learned to use our senses according to the principle buddhi - discriminative intelligence. Specifically, the element earth relates to the thumb and the mount of Venus; water, to the mount and finger of Jupiter; fire, to the mount and finger of Saturn; air, to the mount and finger of Sun; and ether, to the mount and finger of Mercury.*

In the book *Chinese Medical Palmistry*, by Xiao-Fan Zong, various hand shapes are associated with particular elements. For instance, a square-shaped hand is associated with Earth element; a bamboo-shaped hand is associated with Fire element; and a delicately shaped hand is associated with Water element. Thai palmistry is sometimes close to Indian Hast Jyotish palmistry, but usually Thais use Chinese palmistry, which stems from the Indian but is no longer the same. Chinese palmistry is particularly focused on the elements. If you wish to add a divinatory art to your bodywork practice, any of them will do. Palmistry is a natural fit, because it is on the body; it is easier to learn than astrology but not as easy as numerology.

Numerology
Lâyk sàat | เลขศาสตร์

Here is how rampant the significance of numbers is in Thailand: Thai people will often change their phone number simply because they found a sim card with a more auspicious number. This can make maintaining contact with someone more difficult than one would think necessary. In fact, the trend toward insuring a lucky phone number has driven up the price of certain phone numbers in Thailand, with numbers that start with 09 being in particular demand. While a new sim card for a mobile phone in Thailand usually costs only a couple of dollars, very auspicious numbers can be as much as several thousand dollars.

There are several systems of numerology, including Pythagorean numerology (developed by Pythagoras), Chaldean numerology, Kabalistic numerology, Chinese numerology, Indian numerology, and more. Pythagorean, Chaldean, and Kabalistic numerology all work with the characteristics of numbers, whereas Chinese numerology works with the sounds that numbers make and the quality of words that have similar sounds.

Chinese numerology aside, numerology usually works on the idea that a person's name holds a numerical value between one and nine (or one and eight if using Chaldean numerology), and that this number represents qualities inherent in that person. The common form of numerology that most closely resembles Thai numerology is Chaldean. This system uses the name that a person is known by (as opposed to other systems that use the birth name only), taking the letters of the name and adding them up to form a single digit number.

CHAPTER SEVEN

Spirit Medicine

Sǎi-yá-sàa | ไสยศาสตร์

June 8th, 2013, on the bus between Chiang Rai and Chiang Mai

The shaman shack is a raised structure, with concrete steps leading up, made of old thin wood with cracks, and a floor strangely covered in cartoon contact paper. It would take a long time to see everything that is in the room, never mind the small size. The walls are covered in thick, nearly three-dimensional, colorful art pieces—Ganesh, an ascetic, Hanuman, some sort of mystical person with an absolutely three-dimensional penis right about nose level when you sit down on the floor—which is what you do when you are in the shaman shack; you sit. The art is made from medicinal herbs, mashed and dried into thick works of wonder, and painted. The shaman, is an artist.

The altar, jumbled near the ancient television that sometimes shows Thai soaps and the water dispenser, is a clutter of statues, new and dead flowers, incense, herbs, and a large jar with a human fetus floating inside. The fetus is nearly to term. The rest of the room is papers, medicines, bowls, trash bin, tools of the trade, handwritten books of incantations and mantras and magical tattoos, and Reu-sěe da ton poses, whiskey bottles, and dust. Cats and kittens of varying sizes and degrees of tameness wander in and out, and under the shack. An old woman sleeps and putters under there, too.

Shaman isn't actually the right word. The Thai term for this man is maw pii, or "spirit doctor." Most Thai's call him Ajahn, which means "teacher," but not your run-of-the-mill teacher. I'm not sure if we started calling it the Shaman Shack when I first went out there, with a group of five students I was guiding through Thailand, or if the term came about on the next trip, when I took my son Django, day after day, and we discovered that medicine men are not nearly as fascinating to seven-year-olds as they are to adults. I know the term was in use on that trip, though, because I can remember Django saying "Do we have to go to the shaman shack again?" Because really, there are only so many times you can watch people get magical tattoos hammered onto their bodies with a long metal spear. He is unfazed by the blood, the fetus, the dried-out wasp nest. The Thai word for bored, is buaa.

Ajahn makes us breakfast most days that we go out there. Sticky rice, chili eggplant dip, some steamed plants that appear to be weeds, and sometimes eggs laid by the chickens that run around loose at the crematorium down the way. There are frequently other foods that he encourages me to try. Usually something fermented that I am not really so excited about, but he will reassure me that it's vegetarian and wait for the sampling so that he can laugh at my face. This morning, I secretly ate a pancake before going out, just in case gooey fermented bean paste was all that was on the menu. It wasn't the only thing, but it was indeed an option.

Ajahn is my teacher's teacher. He does not speak English, and my Thai cannot keep up with him, so our relationship is mostly just smiles and the occasional comment translated through my teacher, and the tattoos that he has placed forever on my back and arms, and, invisibly, on my leg. They are not aesthetic tattoos, but rather serve various purposes, from protection to connection. They came with chants and rules. I am not allowed to eat star fruit, nor let a man come on the tattoos. The rules are the rules.

If you go to the Shaman Shack, Ajahn might show you his art. Or show you how he can insert a very long nail into his nose. Or show you the other jar, with the smaller fetus inside of it. Or hand you a glass of alcohol. Or make you an amulet for love, money, or protection. Once he gave me a little brass-colored container filled with some sort of special beeswax and a tiny figurine pressed into the beeswax. He told me to smear the wax on my eyebrows and lips when I needed people to like me. Like for a job interview, or when I am teaching. Yes, of course, I have done it; you would too, trust me.

It took me several visits to realize he has a wooden leg from the knee down. My teacher says that he was in a motorbike accident (basically all injuries in Thailand involve the word motorbike) and his leg was badly injured. The doctors could have healed it, but Ajahn could not be bothered with all it would take, so he told them to just cut it off. In Thai, "really" is jing. This is when a Thai person would say "Jing?" and the storyteller would say "Jing jing!"

I feel that I should say more about the fetuses, because I just left them there in the jars, and I think this might be bothering some people. They are not novelties. They are working for Ajahn. The bigger one, the one on the altar, protects his shack. Oh, I should also note that he does not live in this shack. It is his office. I have never seen his house. Anyhow, the bigger fetus, its spirit is protecting the area. My teacher says that no one would dare come mess with Ajahn's shack, not with that kid spirit around. My teacher also says that if you sleep there, you can hear the kid run around and play at night.

The other fetus, the smaller one, is in a jar of some sort of oil. Sometimes, Ajahn will use a bit of the oil for an amulet for someone. So the little fetus, a little part of its spirit, goes off to help that person. Its spirit is scattered, helping various people as needed. Eventually, Ajahn frees the fetus's spirits. They are not made to work for him forever, and it is his job to care for them while they do. Part of that care is in knowing when to release them.

The fetuses come from the bodies of women who died while still pregnant. The husband, or the family, gives Ajahn permission to harvest the unborn babies. In modern Thai hospitals, there is paperwork for this—permission forms for this limping, smiling spirit doctor to come and get the fetus from the mother's body.

He works with the dead a lot. It is his job to care for the bodies at the funeral. He washes them and makes sure that the spirit goes off as it is supposed to. And he burns the bodies, remaining for hours after the family has left, for it takes a long time for a body to burn.

Today, my teacher took me and my friend E. (who is also a student of my teacher) to a funeral. About 75 Thais were gathered outside. Me and E. sat in the back, trying to be *inconspicuous since we didn't know the deceased or his family but, of course, it is not easy for two white-skinned people to be inconspicuous at a Thai funeral.*

There was one other white person attending; I believe he was married to the daughter of the deceased. When all of the offerings and the talking, and the monk moments were done, the white man walked over to us and very kindly asked us what we were doing there. We explained that our teacher's teacher was the medicine man, and the Westerner (who I believe was English), was very warm and did not make us feel like horrible gawkers. He explained, though, that the family sent him over to ask what our story was, figuring that since we were all the same color, he was the best one to do it.

The casket was placed in a furnace, while swirling fireworks went off and the fancy litter that had held the casket until this moment, was lit on fire in a beautiful blaze that we were told cost 26,000 baht, about 800 U.S. dollars. At this point everyone left, except for those whose job it is to attend to the burning body: Ajahn, who peers inside the furnace wielding a long two-pronged pole to turn the body as needed (he tells us that this two-pronged pole is just like the one Hades is depicted with – because Hades also deals with death), and about six men who sit around getting drunk but who will ultimately help with furnace cleanup. The family, to my surprise, does not stay to witness the burning for even a moment. They clear out fast once the casket is on fire, as they believe it is inauspicious to be around this part of death.

E., my teacher, Ajahn, and I gather around the open furnace door to watch the body burn. The serious part of washing the body in the water from a split coconut, and making sure the spirit moves on is done, and now as the body burns, Ajahn jokes about steak and how we are all just meat. It is very, very hot by the open furnace. I am not going to describe the images of the burning corpse; enough to know that it was both horrid and not horrid. It touched me and then again, it did not. Perhaps time will sort this out. I welcomed the whiskey and water on ice that the six drinking men offered though—and I'm not really a whiskey drinker.

At one point, I was staring at the broken coconut sitting on the ground a few feet from the furnace, wondering what would be done with it now, when Ajahn told us that the meat from a coconut used in this ceremony should be eaten by people who grind their teeth at night. The connection seemed random to me, but since Django grinds his teeth, I accepted a portion of it to take home. We ate the spongy palm seed thing that grows inside the mature coconut, and it was only after I swallowed my portion that the impact of eating a coconut whose water just washed a dead body hit me. I was not sure if I liked this bite of coconut inside of me, and I was not sure if I would feed any of it to my child. Uncertain, in Thai, is mai nee jai. It means "not sure in the heart mind."

Ajahn has no prices for the things he does, be it giving amulets, creating tattoos, or presiding over funerals. There are certain works that you can only do for voluntarily donated reciprocation. To set a price on healing, or setting spirits free, would taint the gifts that make him good at these things. Once, we were at the Shaman Shack the day after the funeral of a very poor person, with a very poor family. Ajahn told us that for all his hours of work, they gave him 12 baht, about 50 cents. He laughed and laughed about this. It does not matter; they gave what they could.

I am not important to this medicine man. I am just this person who shows up sometimes with his student. He has, however, literally made a permanent mark on me in a handful of ways. Firstly, as mentioned, he has adorned my body with tattoos. I never had a tattoo before meeting him a handful of years ago, but on the day I met him I let him tattoo my back in ink made of a mixture of ground stones, herbs picked on specific moons, squid ink, and mantras, and applied to the dermis layer of my skin with a long spear-like tool. The Thai word for "tattoo" is sak. Mantra is the spoken sacred symbology. Tantra is the physical sacred symbology. Yantra is the written, or drawn, sacred symbology. So the tattoos that these medicine men create are called sak yan, meaning "tattoo yantra." I did not know what he was putting on my back when he did it, and my teacher waited a full week before telling me the meaning of my new skin. The Thai word for pain is jep.

I have since acquired further sak yan from him, the most recent being the invisible tattoo on my leg. Invisible tattoos are done in a special oil instead of ink, such that once the blood and the wounding heals, nothing is left to see. Thai women, if getting sak yan, tend to go for the invisible.

Ajahn is also the person who initiated me to learn tok sên. The day he initiated me, he made my tok sên tools. He hacked away with a machete, at an old two-by-four that had once been a part of the infrastructure of a Buddhist temple, creating a rough tok sên peg and mallet that are ugly compared to the polished beauties sold at market but are, of course, gorgeous to me. He then wrote mantras on it with a black Sharpie. In Thailand, sacred and practical and mundane all mix together, with no clear lines in between.

So, there are the tattoos, there is the tok sên, there is the experience of spending a little part of my life in a space that most from my part of the world never see, and there is the experience of the burning body. These are the places this man has affected me most obviously. Then there is the fact that he is one of the teachers of the man who has taught me the most about Thai medicine and Buddhism. This is no small thing. But really? I cannot say that I know this man. I am a stranger in a strange land when I am at the Shaman Shack.

I have thought to write about the Shaman Shack a lot over the years, even started to a handful of times, only to let it go, because I don't want to fall into the travelers trap of turning everything into an experience that is almost a commodity, so that even as we are living it, we are planning the Facebook post, the tweet, the blog. Like the funeral: For that family, it was a part of their lives, an end to a life, a moment in time that was theirs. I actually was the gawker that I didn't want to be. I was there to "see a Thai funeral," and to see what a burning body looks like. I was curious, and I was daring myself, because I have some issues with death. I was not there to say goodbye to the dead man, or to comfort those left alive. I was just watching my movie.

So I've not written about the Shaman Shack before, because I worried about turning real life, the sacred, the mystery and the dark, into a travel essay. But you know what?

In Thailand, I have seen monks texting during ceremony. I have been in the Shaman Shack when the television plays soap operas while one person is bowing to the altar and another is receiving a sak yan tattoo while the medicine man is chanting incantations over his work. And Thais take pictures in the temples all the time!

Because in Thailand, the sacred and the mundane and the commercial and the smell of the sewer and the smell of the incense are not separate. The Christians are here in droves converting the ancestor-worshipping animistic Hill Tribe people, but what they do not realize is that to people accustomed to many gods, Christ is more often than not adopted into a family rather than supplanting one. Another god? Fantastic. We can add him to the altar at the mall. It all mixes together.

So here is my travel essay patched together from several years of traipsing out to the Shaman Shack. It's memories and thoughts, and sharing, and yes, turning a window into another life into another experience check mark in the bucket list. See a shaman, get a tattoo, watch a body burn. But because the sacred and mundane don't have to be separate, it's also as real and unreal as anything.

I'm finishing this on the bus heading back down to Chiang Mai. It's been a few weeks since the funeral, and I'll be meeting my teacher back out at the Shaman Shack tomorrow morning for breakfast. I'll stop and eat something not at all scary beforehand so that I don't have to put fetid fermented brown gloppy stuff into an empty stomach. The bus just passed five cars on a blind mountain curve heading downhill. The Thai word for "finished" is set.

Categories (Who is Who)

In order to talk about spirit medicine, I think it will be helpful to talk a bit about the different healing arts roles in Thailand, because it can get a little confusing, especially when we come to spirit medicine. So for starters, I'm going to describe some of the more common roles.

Specialists

Specialists are people who practice a particular healing art, such as *khôodt* (scraping), massage, bone setting, herbalism, and some forms of magic. Traditionally, these roles came with extra responsibilities, in terms of being someone who takes care of their community. Specialists would always have a teacher, and be initiated into a lineage and given initiation to practice their healing art. These days, most massage therapists no longer undergo initiation, as the spa and street massage industry has branched ever farther away from traditions, but technically, anyone practicing Thai massage should get initiated if they have the opportunity. The initiation gives you healing powers and protection.

Initiation is different from ordination, which is what monks undergo. There are rules that go along with healing arts practice and initiations. For example, someone who practices magic might not be allowed to eat certain foods, eat at a funeral, or walk under a banana tree (because there are special ghosts that hang out under banana trees and might attach to them). Those who practice bodywork are expected to hold the precepts, respect their teachers, have a fundamental practice of cultivating the Bhramaviharas, and on the full and new moons they should uphold the eight precepts rather than the standard five (more on the Bhramaviharas and the eight precepts in the section on Buddhism). Depending on their lineage, they may be required to uphold more practices as well.

Specialists receive money for their work; in fact, it is considered important that they be paid, because if there is no reciprocation for this level of healing, it will not work as well. In Thai tradition, patients will generally bring offerings of flowers, incense, and candles, as well as payment for the practitioner. The amount varies, depending on the financial ability of the patient, and those who cannot pay high prices should not be turned away, as the giving is relative to the wealth. There are exceptions to the need for payment though. Monks are never charged for healing services, and usually the elderly are also treated for free. If a therapist offers to treat someone without being asked, then this can be freely given as well. But if the patient requests healing work, then they should pay something for it. Some part of all payments will be donated by the practitioner to their teacher or teachers.

Reu-sĕe / Yogis

reu-sĕe | ฤษี

Reu-sĕes, or yogis, as described earlier, are spiritual ascetics. They are generally solitary researchers and practitioners of the fundamental sciences, such as medicine, geomancy, astronomy and mathematics. Becoming a *Reu-sĕe* is very difficult, as it involves both effort and fate. A *Reu-sĕe* must be ordained into the tradition by a qualified teacher, but ordination will only happen if certain fated events beyond the control of the people involved occur (such as the unsought acquisition of specific objects, such as a bowl, mala, walking stick, text, and animal print cloth).

Ordination is quite serious, preceded by tests and with many precepts that must be upheld, including the Buddhist precepts and often the bodhisattva vow, but cultivation of the brahma-viharas is of primary importance. Different *Reu-sěes* decide to have different levels of contact with lay people. Some may retreat for most of their life; however, at some point, they must record their knowledge or teach others, and medicine *Reu-sěes* must treat those in need. This is one of the many ways in which *Reu-sěe* differ from monks; they have to be able to touch and interact with lay people, including women (in fact, *Reu-sěe* can be female), and it is possible for *Reu-sěe* to marry and have children. While not all *Reu-sěe* spend most of their life in hermitage, they must spend significant amounts of time in nature retreat, as they gain their knowledge and power from the elements and connection to nature, but they must also bring that knowledge back to the community in information and healing.

Reu-sěe counterparts around the world include the shamans of the South Americas, but *Reu-sěe* are Buddhist, so they do not use psychoactive substances in their work; instead, they use meditation to achieve many of the same ends.

Monks
prá sŏng | พระสงฆ์

Monks are Buddhist renunciates who have taken vows to forego the secular way of life. They do not have jobs, nor do they marry, and they do not engage in activities such as listening to music, watching television, or other frivolous pleasures. They uphold strict precepts, and their primary role is to practice the dharma. Many monks also teach lay people who wish to learn the dharma, but some spend their lives in seclusion simply practicing the teachings of the Buddha. Anyone who can commit to upholding the precepts of a monk may be ordained as a *bhikku* (male monk) or *bhikkhuni* (female monk), although there are far less *bhikkhuni* in Thailand.

Mediums
kon song or rang song | คนทรงเจ้า or ร่างทรง

Thai mediums don't channel the dead like Western mediums do; rather, they channel ancestral spirits, teachers of the past, and deities. They are sometimes initiated, and go through a ceremony in which they receive ownership of the deity they are channeling; however, it is not like the other traditions in which a teacher approves you for initiation or ordination, because mediums are chosen by the deity that uses them. They can charge a small fee for their services, but since it is the deity doing the work, not the person, they must donate all of the money they receive (generally to a temple). Keeping the money will lead to unfortunate events. For this reason being a medium is not a job, and they must keep lay person's jobs in order to have an income.

Many mediums are lay people. My teacher describes the four types of mediums, only one of which is real, as follows:

1) **Charlatans** - those who deliberately pretend in order to gain money and fame;
2) **Deluded** - those who are not pretending, but honestly believe that they are mediums, when in fact they are not;

3) **Possessed** - those who are possessed by lower spirits and ghosts who are fooling them and using them for sustenance; and

4) **The real deal.** True mediums are the rarest of the four. I hold this categorization in my mind every time that someone tells me they have any magical or supernatural abilities, as I think that it has application (with the possible exception of number three) to many circumstances.

Spirit Doctors
mŏr pĕe | หมอผี

Now we come to what this chapter is really about. It was important to distinguish the different roles, as the healing the *Reu-sĕes*, specialists, and mediums do can often become confused with spirit doctors. One reason for this confusion is that we do not have a word in English that accurately labels the Thai spirit doctors. We frequently call them medicine men/women, or shamans, but medicine man/woman might as easily apply to an herbalist, and shaman is a bit of an overlap between *Reu-sĕe* and spirit doctors. I use the term "spirit doctor," as this is the literal translation of *mŏr pĕe*, the Thai term for them.

Mŏr pĕe are Buddhist, but they do not hold the precepts of a monk or a *Reu-sĕe*. In fact, their role as a spirit doctor sometimes requires that they engage in behavior that precepts would forbid, such as drinking, and using the darker magics. They work outside of the normal parameters, being kind of the bad boys and girls of healing arts, yet helping many people. They often do things that most lay people, healers, and monks will not or cannot do, such as working directly with spirits and ghosts[74] and handling the dead.

There are spirit doctors, such as the well-known Pichest Boomthame (who is also a bodyworker and a medium), who choose to strictly uphold the Buddhist precepts; however, it is not required of the spirit doctors, and some engage in quite dark activities that would seriously violate precepts.

Mŏr pĕe care for their community in many ways, making magical amulets that protect, heal, or attract (wealth, romance, and so on). They do *sak yan*, the magical tattooing, and they practice spiritual healing techniques such as *yam khan, tok sen, and bplao*. In Thailand it is the *mŏr pĕe*, not the mediums, who channel the dead, as they work directly with spirits. They also ritualistically attend to the bodies of the dead, and make sure that their spirits are set free (and do not hang around to cause troubles). Usually, monks perform a ceremony at the funeral, but they do not interact with the body, and they do not remain once the body is lit on fire.

Yogis will stay during the cremation to meditate on the body, but they also do not usually interact directly with the body.

---

74 Spirits and ghosts are not considered the same thing exactly. A ghost is someone who dies with a last thought attached to something. They die and are reborn as a ghost that is completely attached to that thought. The ghost's life ends when the karma for that is expired, or when they somehow realize what they are doing. Doing offerings for ghosts helps them with this. People can also be reborn as a kind of protective spirit, which has more consciousness than a ghost and can be beneficial or not, depending on events.

Spirit Medicine in a Bodywork Practice

Just as a bodyworker should know enough herbalism to at the very least support the bodywork with balms, poultices, detoxifying teas, and the like, it is important for a bodyworker to incorporate certain aspects of spirit medicine into their work, as Thai medicine is holistic and the five roots all grow into the same tree in whose branches you find your specialty. Here now are some basic spirit medicine practices for a bodywork specialist.

Self-Protection

Thai tradition holds that the most important thing any practitioner can do to protect themselves from taking on any form of suffering from their patient is to do their daily *wai khru* and uphold the five Buddhist precepts. Below is the chant for clearing space and protection.

Recite:

BUDDHAṀ PACCAKKHĀMI

DAMMAṀ PACCAKKHĀMI

SAṄGHAṀ PACCAKKHĀMI

This chant should be repeated seven times after working, to clear the space. For cleansing yourself after a treatment, chant it while washing your hands.

Som Poi / Water

Som poi is a Thai herb that closely resembles dried tamarind pods. In fact, many Westerners who have seen their teachers in Thailand make *som poi* water mistakenly believe that it *is* tamarind. Since the Thai teachers hear their Western students call it this, and don't know that they are mistaken, they think that the English name for *som poi* is tamarind. So now we have Thai massage teachers in Thailand telling their Western students to make tamarind water. It's a small, confusing mess...

In reality, *som poi* is a cleansing herb, used in much the same way that Native Americans in North America use sage, South Americans use *palo santo* wood, and the Chinese use dried orange peel. *Som poi* is not easily found in the West, but I have come across it in our local Thai-run Asian food market, and it can be found for sale online. If you can get some *som poi*, try to have a Thai monk, spirit doctor, or *Reu-sĕe* bless it.

Traditionally, you add fresh kaffir limes and turmeric, recite incantations, and let it all sit for ten to fifteen minutes. Washing your hands in the *som poi* water and sprinkling it on your head will have a cleansing effect, removing toxic energies that you may have taken on while doing healing work.

Healing Incantation

This healing incantation is found in the version of the *wai khru* that is most commonly given to Westerners learning Thai massage in Thailand; however, it is rarely explained to them that it is not a Buddhist verse, but rather, a magical incantation reflective of the spirit medicine root of Thai medicine.

Recite:

OṀ NA-A NA-WA ROGA VYĀDHI VINĀSANTI

You can recite this incantation over those you do healing arts work on, in sets of three recitations. To build your relationship with the incantation you can recite it 108 times regularly, using a mala to keep count. To increase the efficacy of this incantation, recite it daily.

Holy Water

Holy water is given to patients before a treatment, so that while they are receiving bodywork, the water will work on them from the inside out, clearing out any bad energies, spirits, or other unseen negativities. You can also use this water to cleanse yourself. It is easy to make, as you simply recite a couple of verses from your *wai khru* combined with the healing incantation above. You will need the cleanest water you can obtain. Spring water is ideal, but not the kind that comes in plastic bottles, as this contains plastic contaminants and is injurious to our planet.

After your regular practice of *wai khru*, make offerings of flowers, candles, and incense as you bring the water to your altar space. The water is ideally in a glass or copper bowl, but any natural material will do (no plastic or aluminum). You can place a crystal in the water while you charge it if you like.

Recite over the water:

NAMO TASSA BHAGAVATO ARAHATO SAMMA SAMBUDDHASSA (3 TIMES)
OṀ NA-A NA-WA ROGA VYĀDHI VINĀSANTI *(7, 9, or 12 times)*

Blow on the water, then recite:

METTĀ GUṆAṀ ARAHAṀ METTĀ *(3 times)*

Blow on the water again, and the process is complete.

You can give a cup of this water to your patients before you work on them. You don't have to tell them anything about it, as it will just be water to them, but you can watch for the subtle changes it may bring. Just know that they will most likely be subtle indeed, and don't expect big dramatic shifts. You may simply notice that people are more relaxed, or that they report an extra good experience. At my house, we find that holy water takes on a faint vanilla flavor.

Another way to make holy water is to chant the homage to Jīvaka Kumārabhacca from the *wai khru* 108 times with a mala. Allow the end of the mala to hang into the water, so that the beads cycle through the water (of course, wash your hands first, since you will be touching each bead that will then touch the water).

Kwǎn String
Sòo kwǎn | สู่ขวัญ

When you travel in Thailand, there is a strong chance that you will at some point find yourself having a string tied around your wrist by a teacher, a monk, or a host. These strings are called *kwǎn* strings, and they are used to bless your *kwǎn*. Some say that the string blessing helps to tie your *kwǎn* to you, so that it will not leave you. *Kwǎn* strings are usually given at important times in life, such as a baby's first ceremonial tonsure (hair cutting), graduation from a course of study, weddings, and prior to going on a journey. Anyone can give someone a *kwǎn* string, and they are often given by parents and teachers. On this level it is a simple blessing. When given by a spirit doctor or a monk, the blessing is considered much stronger and magical.

To give someone a *kwan* string blessing, tie a piece of plain soft cotton string around their wrist and recite the following verses.

BUDDHAṀ PASIDDHI DHAMMAṀ PASIDDHI SAṄGHAṀ PASIDDHI
BUDDHAṀ RAKKHAṀ DHAMMAṀ RAKKHAṀ SAṄGHAṀ RAKKHAṀ

Spirit Medicine Practices

Yam kǎang | ยํ่าขาง

Yam kǎang is a spirit medicine technique used for ridding a patient of evil spirits, ghosts, and black magic. The doctor first puts the bottom of his foot in oil (usually herbal oil) and then quickly touches his foot to a red hot metal (usually a piece of a plow that has been heating over hot coals), often causing flames to briefly fly up around his foot. He then places his foot on the problem area of the patient. I use the male gender pronoun here because traditionally women do not practice *yam kǎang* due to an increased risk of spiritual possession. This is connected to women having receptive energy, while men have sending energy. Hence, we see a male practitioner casting out negative influences from the patient's body.

Like a few other spirit medicine techniques, *yam kǎang* has started to gain interest from non-Thais these days, and is beginning to be taught as a massage technique. I cannot stress enough that *yam kǎang* is *not* a massage modality; it is spirit medicine for working with negative influences of a spiritual nature and for driving out spirits, and if you have not been initiated and trained in a spirit medicine lineage, it will not be an effective healing technique—instead, it will feel like a slimy damp foot pressing on the body with no real purpose, because the effectiveness of *yam kǎang* does not come from the physical actions involved. The physical actions are a vehicle for the magic.

Chét & hâek | เช็ดแฮก

Chét & hâek are healing techniques that involve reciting magical healing incantations over the patient while gently rubbing them with a special tool, or sweeping their body with a leaf, string, or your hand. *Chét* involves lighter sweeping motion, while *hâek* involves slightly stronger contact. They are not the same, but you often hear the term *chét hâek* used together, almost as if it were one word.

I've seen a number of *chét hâek* tools and they have each been unique. Once, a traditional medicine practitioner in northern Thailand showed me his collection of *chét hâek* tools, and they made me think of a magpie's treasure. A rock, a boar's tusk, an old piece of metal—precious items that would not generally be recognized as such. What all of the *chét hâek* tools I've seen have had in common was that they were old, and had been given to the practitioner by his or her teacher.

Chét hâek is good to do after other treatments, as it removes all sorts of residual problems with spirit and *kwăn*, and it can also help to rid the patient of any strong mental fixation or attachment to the ailment that might be getting in the way of healing. It does this because it affects the *kwăn*, and *kwăn* is related to the connection between the body and the mind. *Chét hâek* also helps if there is black magic, or if we have unintentionally inherited a spirit that is attached to a used item we have bought or been gifted, and it is good for mystery pain. It is also used for injuries and diseases. *Chét hâek* comes from Lanna culture.

Bpào | เป่า

Bpào is essentially just like *chét hâek,* only without the tools. Instead of using a tool to get the magic in, the incantations are blown into the patient. The spirit doctor recites the incantations and then blows on the patient's skin.

Jòp kài | จอบไข่

Jòp kài is another kind of magical healing technique that draws out poisons, black magic, spirits, and ghosts. There are two types of *jòp kài*, both of which use an egg to draw out the negative influences. In one form of *jòp kài,* a raw egg is rubbed on the patient while the spirit doctor recites specific incantations. When the egg is cracked open afterwards, various objects may be found inside, such as dirt, old nails, really anything.

In the second form of *jòp kài,* an old coin is wedged inside a boiled egg. The egg is then wrapped in a cloth, and again the egg is rubbed on the patient, with the doctor speaking incantations. When the coin is removed from the egg it will have changed color to varying degrees. It might be green or black or brown. This coin will be cleaned and then used again on other patients. I have seen the same coin turn a variety of colors depending on the patient. Because of the variance in the results of both of these forms of *jòp kài,* they are diagnostic as well as therapeutic.

Using eggs to heal, cleanse, and detoxify the body is a practice that can be found in many places around the world. The *curanderas* of South America, the Catholic Benedicaria of Italy, and the Romani of Spain all have their forms of egg cleansing. Egg healing is also rather notorious for being used by charlatans, so be careful!

Sàk yan | สักยันต์

Sàk yan is spiritual or magical tattooing. It is done for many different purposes, depending on the desire of the patient. Protective *sàk yan* is very popular with people who are in dangerous professions, such as law enforcement or the military, but *sàk yan* can also be used for connection to deities, wisdom, compassion, and any number of things. The ink for *sàk yan* is made from a mixture of medicinal plants, minerals, and squid ink, and all ingredients are gathered under particular moons, with incantations and ceremony. It is said to be very powerful stuff.

Traditionally, *sàk yan* is applied with a long, spearlike tool that the spirit doctor repeatedly stabs the patient's skin with. *Sàk* is the Thai word for "tattoo," and *yan* comes from the Sanskrit word *yantra,* which means "the spoken or drawn sacred symbology." If you go to Thailand and you wish to get *sàk yan*, make sure that you get it from a qualified practitioner. There are street tattoo artists who give tattoos that look like *sàk yan*, but are not the real thing.

Tok Sên | ตอกเส้น

Tok Sên is a healing arts modality from Lanna culture that uses a heavy wooden mallet called a *káwn*, and a light wooden peg called a *lîm* (the wood for these tools is considered best if it comes from a lightning-struck tree or the wood from an old temple). The mallet is used to strike the peg, which is in contact with the body of the treatment recipient. This is a powerful dispersing technique, a little like beating turned all the way up. It is used to treat the *sên* by tapping directly on the *sên*, or on the trenches.

Tok sên is beneficial for blockages, stagnation, paralysis, and poor circulation. It can chase poisons in the body to a specific point from which the body can be bled if there is a therapist qualified to do so. It aids the flow of wind (movement) in the body, can treat sickness as well as relaxing the *sên* and muscles. It is very good for people with dense tissue, because it penetrates deeply but is a gentle therapy, and it is much easier than using your hands when the tissue is very dense.

Tok sên is an overlap modality between spirit medicine and physical therapies. Unlike *yam kǎang*, the purely physical efficacy of *tok sên* is clear, and I struggled in deciding which chapter I should put *tok sên* in. Ultimately, I chose spirit medicine because it is very important that this side of the art not be forgotten. It is traditionally only taught to those who have participated in an initiation ceremony with a teacher qualified to initiate. This teacher will also bless the *tok sên* tools to empower them and give the student incantations to be used in conjunction with *tok sên* healing.

It is considered dangerous and inappropriate to learn and practice *tok sên* without proper initiation, as the practitioner becomes vulnerable to taking on the patient's illness and spirits/ghosts that may be lingering around the patient. Different incantations are used in different lineages, and it is necessary to receive the incantations directly from the mouth of a teacher, not from a printed text. If you have received *tok sên* incantations, you should not share them with others.

These days, *tok sên* is becoming popular with Western Thai massage therapists, who are frequently learning only the technique, without initiation, incantations, or any medical theory. This last part alone is rather dangerous, as *tok sên* can break bones and should not be used randomly. Also, it is now being taught as a massage treatment for the whole body, when traditionally, it was just a spot-specific therapy that was primarily done in conjunction with other massage techniques, or *chet* and *hâek*. A good progression would be to use massage techniques to assess and soften the body, then use *tok sên*, and follow up with *chét hâek*.

Tok sên is a truly amazing and effective therapy, but finding teachers who are qualified to pass on initiation and incantations is becoming ever harder as the older generations, who subscribed more readily to traditional medicine, are dying out. It is still possible, though, and if you have the chance to become initiated I highly recommend it. At the time of this writing, I myself am not qualified to initiate students, so I practice but do not teach this therapy, out of respect for my teachers and in honor of traditions.

Finally, in addition to having an incantation or two at your disposal, you can round out your bodywork practice by being able to refer your patients to local people who can fill the role that spirit medicine fills in Thailand. This might mean sending them to their priest, a Native American medicine man/woman, a *curandera*, a Hawaiian *kahuna*, or a Jewish rabbi. People in all cultures and traditions have someone who takes on the work of attending to their community's spiritual healing, and since it is very hard for Westerners to get training in Thai spirit medicine, we can look elsewhere for what will best benefit our individual patients.

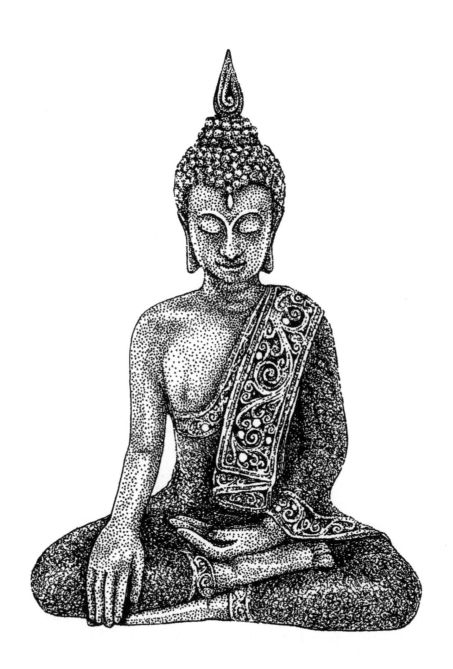

CHAPTER EIGHT

Buddhism

Pút-tá-sàat | พุทธศาสตร์g

Buddhism and medicine fit together. Buddhism, the Dharma, is throughout medicine. It's one of the 5 roots of medicine, so it pervades everything, starting with the view and how we view the body and how we view disease, how we view phenomena, and how we view nature. This all comes from Buddhism. How we understand the body in terms of elements, how we understand the functions of the body and the disease-causing factors of the elements. This all is coming from the Dharma. The view comes from the understanding of the body from the Buddhist perspective. And then, of course, ethics, our approach to diagnostics and treatment, all of this is coming from the Buddha's teachings. It's pretty much pervasive in Thai medicine, or any traditional medicine from the Buddhist traditions.

— *TEVIJJO YOGI*

Buddhism and Medicine

As I have said, while not all Buddhist medicine is Thai medicine, Thai medicine is inherently Buddhist medicine. It maintains the ancient flavors of Animism, and is influenced by many cultures, but at its heart, it is Buddhist medicine with a Thai spin. The main branches of Buddhism are Theravada, Mahayana, and Vajrayana Buddhism. They all contain the same core teachings of the Buddha, but the different branches have different teachings that they focus on more. Generally, they are harmonious with one another, and not in dispute. The branch of Buddhism that is mainly practiced in Thailand is Theravada Buddhism, known as the oldest form.

When you really look closely you can see that Thai medicine is rooted in the dharma. You have already been learning the Buddha's teachings throughout this book, as you learn medical theory. In the *Dhatu Vibhanga Sutta*, the Buddha is recorded as saying:

Man consists of six element, six spheres of contact, eighteen mental ramblings, and four resolutions ... The elements are Earth, Water, Fire, Wind, Space, and Consciousness ... What is Earth element? There is internal and external Earth element. What is internal Earth element? It is the hard, internal personal Earth element. What is internal earth element? It is the hard, internal, personal Earth, such as hair on the head, on the body, nails, teeth, outer skin, flesh, veins, bones, bone marrow, kidney, heart, liver, lungs, spleen, intestines, larger intestines, belly, excreta, and many other things that are hard, internal, personal and fixed as one's own. This internal and external earth is the earth element. These are not me. I'm not them. They are not self. This should be seen with right wisdom, as it really is and the mind should be nipped and detached from the Earth element.

What is the Water element? There is internal and external Water element. What is internal Water element? That which is internal, personal, watery, and fixed as one's own, such as bile, phlegm, pus, blood, sweat, oil of the body, tears, oil of the eyes, spit, snot, oil of the joints, urine, and any other thing that is internal, personal, watery and fixed as one's own ... This is internal Water element. This internal Water element and the external Water element, go as Water element. These are not me. I am not in them. They are not self. This should be seen with right wisdom, as it really is and the mind should be nipped and detached from the Water element.

He then continues to explain each of the elements as he explained Earth and Water, and as you have learned them already in this book. And so we begin to see that a meditation on the elements is a meditation on the dharma.

To truly study Buddhism, I recommend that you find a good teacher. There are many wonderful books on Buddhism, but interpretations of the dharma can be confusing, and when one begins to meditate it is good to have guidance. Also, the way that Sanskrit/Pali translates into English can sometimes be off-putting to new students, or at least it was for me. Having a qualified teacher to answer the questions that will arise is beneficial and gentles the learning experience.

In this chapter, I'm going to give a rough outline of some of the Buddha's core teachings, but since I know that some of you will drop off in the reading on Buddhism, I'll begin with most essential practices for a medicine practitioner and then move into the core teachings.

Meditations on The Elements

Knowledge of the elements is key to understanding Traditional Thai Medicine. So far we have approached this on an academic level, which is a good place to start, but intellectualizing the elements will only provide us with a certain level of understanding. Experience working with people and viewing the world through the lens of everything being made of elements is essential for deeper understanding, as is contemplation and meditation.

Earth

To meditate on the Earth element, sit directly on the earth (this can be dirt, grass, floor, and so on). The mantra *Paṭhavī kasiṇaṁ* can be chanted with a mala,[75] and being in the earth, like in a cave, or covered with sand, will also connect you to the Earth element. Contemplate the raw element. This means thinking of Earth in the form of clay, or the desert floor, boulders, things like this. Contemplate the experience of Earth element, which is solidity. Contemplate the nature of solidity. If seeking connection with the Earth element, one should meditate on this element for twenty days.

---

75 A mala is a string of 108 beads (or a division of 108) that is used as a counting tool while chanting.

Water

The mantra for Water is *Āpo kasiṇaṁ*. To connect with the Water element, meditate on water for twelve days, and put yourself near water, such as a pond, a large bowl of water, or a puddle. Contemplate water in its raw form. Contemplate the experience of water, which is aqueousness. Contemplate the nature of fluidity. Unless trying to connect with the Earth element, one should always sit on a mat or cushion when doing element meditations.

Fire

To meditate on the Fire element, put yourself near the external element of Fire, be it a candle, the sun, or a fireplace fire, and chant the mantra *Tejo kasiṇaṁ* with a mala. Contemplate fire in its raw form, and the experience of fire, which is heat. Fire should be meditated on for four days. Unless trying to connect with the Earth element, one should always sit on a mat or cushion when doing element meditations.

Wind

To connect with the Wind element, chant the mantra *Vāyo kasiṇaṁ* with a mala, and put yourself in windy places, such as mountaintops, river gorges, and beaches. Contemplate wind in its raw form, blowing. Contemplate the experience of the Wind element, which is movement. To connect with the Wind element, meditate on it for six days. Unless trying to connect with the Earth element, one should always sit on a mat or cushion when doing element meditations. When learning about and connecting to the elements, it is best to begin with Earth, and move up from heaviest to lightest. Beginning with the Wind element can cause problems in your body and mind.

The Brahmaviharas

The *Brahmaviharas*, also known as the Sublime Attitudes, the Four Immeasurables, or the Divine Abodes, are the qualities, or virtues, that the Buddha encouraged all people to cultivate within themselves and to spread throughout the world. These qualities are *mettā* (loving-kindness), *karunā* (compassion), *muditā*, (sympathetic joy), and *upekkhā* (equanimity). It is extremely important for practitioners of medical science to generate these qualities, as they are necessary in order to be a good practitioner, and also because they are the antidote to the suffering caused by greed, hatred, and ignorance.

Beyond this, the *brahmaviharas*, not money or fame, should be the motivation to help people. Things like compassion and loving-kindness do not provide the healing itself—for that, you must study medicine; but they do provide the impetus to heal, and this is vitally important.

Mettā

At a Buddhist temple in Portland, Oregon, where an old Thai monk named Ajahn Fa Thai gives dharma talks, I once heard him say the following:

Wherever you are, it is a good idea to try to make wishes for people you see. You can do it while you are a passenger in a car, like if you see someone, anyone, just try to think of a little wish for them. If you don't know anything about them you can just think "I wish that they will be happy." But if you can, look for a specific wish you can make for them. When I lived in Thailand there was a little boy who I would see all the time who had very big ears. I would think "I wish that the other children will not tease him for having big ears." Once I saw a woman wearing very high heels and I thought "I wish for her to get sensible shoes so her feet will be comfortable." See, it doesn't have to be hard. You can just make small wishes for people.

Without saying it directly, he was teaching about *mettā*. *Mettā* is usually translated as loving-kindness, or goodwill. *Metta* is the sincere wish for all beings to be peaceful and well. *Mettā* is concern for others. *Mettā* is friendliness. It is the renunciation of animosity, and the true, unselfish desire for the well-being of others. With *mettā*, we see that person over there is just another person like me, so be kind. *Mettā* is associated with the element of Wind.

All of the *Brahmaviharas* have what is called "a near enemy" and "a far enemy." The far enemies are obvious, but the near enemies can trick us; we can think that we are embodying a *Brahmavihara* when really we are not. The near enemy of *mettā* is selfish affection. An example of this would be a parent or a lover who thinks that they are expressing loving-kindness when, in fact, they are only seeking their own joy through the presence of another. The far enemy of *mettā* is painful ill will. This one is easy to see and cannot be confused with *mettā*.

In a healing arts practice, it is necessary to strive to have goodwill toward all, for a doctor cannot go about picking and choosing who they wish to aid. For this reason, healing arts practitioners must cultivate *metta*. Cultivation of the *Brahmaviharas* generally begins with oneself and those in your immediate sphere of affection, and then expands to include all beings, moving from what is easy to what is not as easy. A classic *mettā* meditation might look like this:

May I be peaceful and happy and well;
May my friends and family be peaceful and happy and well;
May those who are suffering in this world be peaceful and happy and well;
May those who cause suffering in this world be peaceful and happy and well;
May all beings on this earth be peaceful and happy and well;
May all beings throughout the universes, and in realms known and unknown,
be peaceful and happy and well.

This is the basic format for many meditations on the Brahmaviharas. Another approach is to begin close and work your way out. For instance, wishing goodwill to everyone in the room with you, then expanding that wish to convey goodwill to everyone in the building, then the block, the neighborhood, the town, the state/province/county, the country, the continent, the planet, the everything. Beginning with self is important. If you are very angry, it can be difficult to feel *mettā* toward others. But if you begin by feeling *mettā* toward yourself, then it becomes possible to offer it outward.

Karunā (Garunā)

Karunā is compassion. It is feeling empathy for those who are suffering. *Karunā* understands that we all suffer in this life, and kindly cares when it sees the suffering. Anyone who has ever experienced a doctor who lacks compassion can tell you in a flash that compassion is needed in the medical sciences. In *Medicine and Compassion: A Tibetan Lama's Guidance for Caregivers* by Chokyi Nyima Rinpoche, Donald Fineberg, Erik Pema Kunsang, and David Shlim, the authors write:

> *The same qualities of mind that foster compassion—tolerating uncertainty, moment-to-moment awareness, openness to new information—can also engender better clinical decision making. Compassion promotes competence. Compassionate physicians stay better focused on the true needs of their patients, while taking full advantage of expert knowledge in treating them. This way, compassion directly expresses patient-centered care, a key constituent of high-quality health care.*

Karunā must be tempered with wisdom, or else you may give away all that you have. This might be compassionate toward others, but it is not compassionate to yourself. The element associated with *Karunā* is Water, and the near enemy of *Karunā* is pity. This is the one that will fool you, as we can easily think we are being compassionate when actually we are being pitying. While everyone needs compassion, no one wants to be pitied. The far enemy of Karunā is cruelty.

Mudita

Mudita is sympathetic joy. This means feeling happiness for the health, wealth, happiness, and success of others. It genuinely celebrates the well-being of others, regardless of your own current situation. *Mudita* sees that happiness begets happiness and wishes for all the world to be happy. In the healing arts, we can see also that doctors must have joy for the well-being of their patients, even if it means they will not be profiting from suffering. *Mudita* is associated with the element of Fire. Its near enemy is exuberance. This can be a bit hard for some to understand, but extreme joy is not considered healthy in the dharma. Extreme joy is unsustainable and leads to the suffering of its passing. It is like a drug that people crave and cling to. Balanced happiness, while less romantic, perhaps, is what *mudita* is about. The far enemy of *mudita* is jealousy or resentment. It can be useful, when you have feelings of jealousy, to simply say to yourself *"mudita."*

Uppekha

Uppekha is about balance, and it is associated with the element of Earth. It is about not seeing the differences in people due to race, money, gender, or education, and it is also about not seeing the differences between beings. *Uppekha* understands that we all have the same potential for enlightenment and suffering. When one cultivates *Uppekha*, one becomes more steady and balanced, and less easily influenced by things such as insults or compliments. *Uppekha* is also about understanding that everyone has their own karma in play, and we must accept this.

When we cultivate *Uppekha* we strive to treat all beings and situations with equality; we learn to let each thing be as it is, and we develop an even and still mind in all circumstances. For a medicine practitioner, this can mean not melting down if you cannot save a patient. It is not beneficial to the patient or their family and other loved ones if the doctor is unbalanced and emotionally caught up.

You must be careful, though, because the near enemy of *Uppekha* is indifference. It is a very common mistake made by people who begin to study Buddhism, to think that to be Buddhist means that they must be unattached to the point of indifference. They become cold and un-emotional. The problem with this is that it leads to suffering, and also it forgets the other three *Brahmaviharas*. For you cannot be indifferent while maintaining goodwill, compassion, and shared joy. The far enemy of *Uppekha* is craving and clinging.

One last thought about the Brahmaviharas. It has become popular with Western Thai massage therapists to use the word *mettā* almost as a catchphrase. I see online posts in which people talk about how much *mettā* they infuse their practice with, and people sign letters "with *mettā*." I understand the sentiment, and I see that what is behind it is an embracing of something love-ly, but I also see how we easily replace actions with words. I once saw a Western Thai massage therapist sign a letter that was threatening a lawsuit, "with *mettā*." What I want to instill here is the understanding that cultivating the *Brahmaviharas* is internal work. Loving-kindness isn't expressed by saying "I have loving-kindness."

If we meditate on loving-kindness, and strive every day to cultivate it, and take the time to notice when we are unkind, we will not need to announce our *mettā*, as it will be clear enough on its own. Having others see you as perfecting loving-kindness should not be the motivation, anyhow; the motivation ought to simply be that we know a world in which humans treat other living beings with good will, is a healthier world for all. Knowing this, we each strive to do our part to create it by nourishing awareness of good-will within ourselves.

The same goes for each of the *Brahmaviharas*. When we eat healthy food and drink healthy fluids, we don't go around telling everyone. Our bodies process the goodness from within and use it to form a clearly healthy being. Make the *Brahmaviharas* internal work, and the nourish-ment from them will radiate off you without need for words, other than the words of kindness that come naturally from this work.

Dedications of Merit

In Buddhist countries, there is an idea that as we go through our days and our lives we accumu-late merit through small and large acts of goodness. Merit is kind of like a protective, beneficial karma. This merit is thought to benefit us in this life, and perhaps in other lives. When you dedicate your merit, you give away whatever merit you gained that day, whether you were aware of doing good or not, to others. You can simply give it away for the good of all, or you can give it to someone you know who is in need, or you can give it to the benefit of someone who has died. Dedicating merit is another way of bringing healing to others, and is a lovely practice for medicine workers.

Some say that you should not give away your merit, because then you will have none, but my teacher says that it does not work this way, and his words ring true for me. He says that while this should not be the motivation behind it, the very act of dedicating merit gains you more merit.

To dedicate your merit, fill a small vessel with water and have an empty vessel at hand. Recite the following verse while pouring the water from one vessel into the other. When you are done, pour the water out onto the earth. Usually people try to pour it out by a tree or other plant. This verse is already in the *wai khru* ceremony given at the beginning of this book, but I wanted to provide it with a bit more focus here.

> *Idam Me Dānam Āsavakkhayāvaham Hotu*
> *Idam Me Sīlam Nibbānassa Paccayo Hotu*
> *Idam Me Bhāvanam Maggassa Ca Phalassa Ca Paccayo Hotu*
> *Idam Me Punnam Āsavakkhayāvaham Nibbānam Hotu*
> *Idam Me Punna Bhāgam Sabba Sattānam Dema*

The Four Noble Truths

The Four Noble Truths were taught in the Buddha's first talk after becoming enlightened, and he continued to give teachings on them throughout his life. They are the foundation, or the framework, for everything else in the dharma.

The First Noble Truth

The first noble truth acknowledges that life is filled with suffering (*dukkha*). In this truth is an understanding that all people everywhere, regardless of class or race or gender, will experience suffering in this life. Everyone will lose a loved one, become injured, become ill, and become old. This is not a fatalistic view that sees nothing but the negative; it is a realistic view that recognizes the fact that life involves suffering. Of course, life also involves pleasure, but this is not a problem in the way that suffering is.

The Second Noble Truth

The second noble truth recognizes that we know the cause of suffering, and this cause is attachment to desire. There are three kinds of desire: 1) **Desires of the sense organs**— cravings for tastes, touch sensations, sounds, and so on; 2) **Desires of becoming**—wanting to become wealthy, wanting to become happy, wanting to become smarter, a better meditator, a more powerful person, enlightened, and so on; and 3) **Desires of unbecoming**—wanting to be rid of anger or bad habits, or wanting to not feel pain. The cause of suffering is also worded as thirsting or craving.

The Third Noble Truth

The third noble truth recognizes that it is possible to end suffering. This states that by understanding the existence of suffering and its causes, we can bring about the cessation of suffering.

The Fourth Noble Truth

The fourth noble truth states that the cessation of suffering can be brought about by following the Noble Eightfold Path. The Four Noble Truths are often likened to medicine, with the Buddha being the physician. In the first noble truth, he identifies the disease (suffering). In the second noble truth, he identifies the cause of the disease. In the third noble truth, he tells the patient that there is hope, that they can get well. And in the fourth noble truth, he gives the prescription of the Noble Eightfold Path.

The Noble Eightfold Path

This, then, is The Buddha's prescription for well-being. It consists of eight things that must be accomplished. They are not done in sequence, one after the other, but are rather all a part of a harmonious life.

1. Right View

Right view is also called right understanding. This is the ability to see things clearly. To understand the true nature of things. It is also understanding the Four Noble Truths. With right view, we see things as they really are, with objectivity and discernment. The most beneficial step you can take toward cultivating right view is to meditate.

2. Right Intention

With right view, we are able to see that which we need to change within ourselves. We can see our angers and jealousies, we can see how we need to develop compassion and loving-kindness, and we can see the difference between right and wrong. With right view to guide us, we aspire toward right intention. Right intention, also called right thought, or right resolve, is the resolution to drive out malefic ways of being and to cultivate beneficial ways of being.

3. Right Speech

With right speech, we resolve to use our words with kindness and compassion, and to not engage in false, divisive, and unkind speech and not to engage in idle chatter.

4. Right Action

Right action is also known as right conduct. It involves striving to abstain from harmful actions, such as killing, stealing, and adultery.

5. Right Livelihood

Right livelihood advises against engaging in businesses that cause harm. There are five livelihoods that the Buddha specifically advised against partaking in.
    These are:
- Dealing in weapons
- Dealing in human beings, such as prostitution and slave trading
- Dealing in the slaughter of animals, including animal husbandry for meat production

and the sale of meat
- Dealing in the trade of intoxicants, such as alcohol and drugs (exception being for medicinal treatment)
- Dealing in poison

6. Right Effort

Right effort is the cultivation of the positive qualities of the mind. This involves nourishing generosity and compassion and freeing oneself from things like aversion and hatred.

7. Right Recollection

Right recollection is also known as right mindfulness, and right memory. Here we recall our practice, and all that we are supposed to do. We keep awareness of, and bring to mind, all of the other parts of the eightfold path, such as our view and thought and intention. In addition, we recall all of the good qualities that we are trying to bring forth.

8. Right Concentration

Right concentration is a perfection of meditation. It is the realization of that which we strive for, be it letting go of ego clinging or achieving understanding of non-self.

The Three Characteristics

The Three Characteristics were taught by the Buddha as being universal to all sentient beings. They are the characteristics of impermanence, suffering, and non-self.

Impermanence

Impermanence, or *anicca*, is the reality that it is the nature of all things to change. This is a core point of the Buddha's teachings. Everything evolves, ripens, dissolves, ends, fluctuates, moves, and passes. A mountain or a building are as impermanent as happiness or sorrow. Even before the eons cause the mountain to erode into a valley, it is changed with each season and passing cloud. Nothing is permanent.

Suffering

Suffering, or *dukkha*, is directly connected to impermanence as it is our attachment to things not changing that creates occasion for suffering. We wish to hold onto our youth, our health, a happy emotion, a person, or an object, but since all things change, we cannot. Suffering is mitigated through the cessation of ignorance, craving, and clinging.

Non-Self

Non-self, or *anatta*, is the Buddha's teaching of the nonexistence of a soul or a single defining object that is "I". While Buddhism recognizes reincarnation, it does not include the idea of a continuous soul entity but rather holds that we are a collection of aggregates, or factors, and that reincarnation is more a result of a force from one lifetime to the next than it is a traveling of an ethereal being from body to body. Reincarnation has been likened to the inherited motion of one billiard ball from the impact of another billiard ball, or to the lighting of one flame from another, as when we light a candle from the flame of a different candle.

Buddhism and the Causes of Suffering

In addition to the many causes of imbalance listed in the Disease and Imbalance chapter, Buddhism, and therefore Thai medicine, contains the understanding that ultimately suffering is caused by desires, as mentioned in The Four Noble Truths, and by mental afflictions called *kilesas*. *Kilesas* are thought and emotion patterns of anger, jealousy, greed, attachment, apathy, pride, and other negative states that cause suffering within oneself and others. All *kilesas* are said to stem from the Three Poisons: attachment, aversion, and ignorance. The Three Poisons are considered to be the root of all evil, toxins that poison the mind.

Attachment

This poison is also known as greed. It is the always wanting, clinging, and craving of desire—attachment to wealth, to a state of being, to an ideology, or to another person. Attachment is the poison of Wind element. It is healed by acts of generosity and by cultivating *uppehkkā*, equanimity.

Aversion

Aversion is also known as anger. This poison embodies hatred and aggression but also resentment, wounded pride, and poisonous jealousy. Aversion is the poison of Fire element. The antidote is practicing *mettā*, loving-kindness.

Ignorance

Ignorance is not knowing, not having Right View, believing in the possibility of permanence, and not understanding The Four Noble Truths. Ignorance does not see the illusion in the world. It feeds the other two poisons of aversion and greed, for one must be in a state of ignorance to believe that greed and anger are worthy states of being. Ignorance is the poison of Water element. The antidote is wisdom. Wisdom is acquired through effort, meditation, and study of the dharma.

Karma and Medicine

In the long run, all of our diseases, injuries, imbalances, and other forms of suffering can be attributed to karma (happiness, as well, but since this is about medicine we'll stick to what needs fixing). Karma is not about punishment and reward, but is simply the natural consequence of our volitional thoughts, words, and deeds in this life and in past lives.

For the most part, we address medicine in terms of seeing fairly direct cause and effect, such as too much spice and sun leads to a Fire imbalance, or not paying attention leads to a car crash and resulting injuries. We can see these things and treat as needed. Knowing the karma that may be behind them is beyond the abilities of most lay people, so we leave it to those whose work it is to touch upon deeper sight and understanding. But there are a couple of areas in medicine in which karma comes into play that bear mentioning here.

First, the unresolved suffering. The shoulder that has always hurt and no doctor can figure out why. The chronic illness that has no cure. The pathological depression that no amount of love and health and wealth can chase away. We go from doctor to doctor, from biomedicine to herbs, from herbs to sweat lodges, and from sweat lodges to books on the power of positive thinking, but we do not get better.

Eventually, it may be determined that the suffering is a karmic occurrence that simply must play itself out. But karma is tricky, for those of us who are not seers cannot know when or how or if the karma will complete in this life. It may be that the next herb you try will be a part of the karmic healing, so complete passivity may not be advisable. Sometimes though, with ongoing suffering, there can be relief in coming to the conclusion that it just has to be, and the questing for a cure can, if not cease, at least relax.

Second, there is often a karmic relationship between healing arts practitioners and patients. Sometimes, it doesn't matter how much skill and knowledge a medical worker has, they just cannot help the person. It may even be someone who has a completely curable imbalance, one that the doctor is particularly talented at fixing—if that doctor is not the karmic healer for that person they will not be able to be of assistance, although they may point the way toward the answer.

This is also why sometimes a skillful doctor may fail to help someone who turns around and is then healed by a complete charlatan. In this case, the charlatan had a karmic healing relationship with the patient, and actual knowledge was not the primary factor. Because of this, we have to be aware of when we are not helping people. Don't hang on to the desire to be the one who solves the problem overly long; instead, be open to helping people to move along and find the right healer for them.

Regarding Becoming Buddhist

One does not have to "become Buddhist" in order to study and benefit from the *dharma*. It is not like some religions, where one must prove oneself or accept one God over all others. It's not about if you meditate, or if you study the *dharma* a certain length of time. What is important is that you find truth in the Four Noble Truths and the Three Characteristics. Taking refuge in the teachings of the Buddha, meaning that you find solace in the *dharma*, is also important. If you wish to join a *sangha*, a Buddhist community, you will probably engage in an official refuge-taking ceremony.

The Buddha was not a god in the sense of other religious figureheads, so Buddhism is not in conflict with other religions. It does not seek to supplant another spiritual teacher or path, and in Thailand, where most people are Buddhist, you find shrines to Hindu gods and goddesses everywhere, with no thought of disharmony or incongruity.

Many Westerners like to approach Buddhism as a philosophy, or simply good advice for a peaceful harmonious life, and leave any sense of religious associations out of it. In Thailand,

and most of Asia, it most definitely has a strong religious feeling to it, but the Buddha wanted the *dharma* to be accessible everywhere, so putting it into a context that is more gentle for Westerners, such as philosophy, does not go against the original teachings.

So for you dear readers, I invite you to cultivate *mettā*, to meditate, and to seek to see the world through awake and open eyes. But you do not have to engage with Buddhism in any way that is uncomfortable to you in order to practice Thai medicine. You only have to understand the teachings.

The Precepts

The most basic and fundamental action undertaken in Buddhism is to aspire to uphold the Five Precepts. These precepts are in the *wai khru* ceremony presented at the beginning of this book, and will be elaborated on here.

1. The Precept to Abstain from Killing

This is a vow made to oneself to not engage in activities that harm or kill any living being. This precept has a flip side, in that it is also a vow to help any being that you can help. As a medicine worker, it is a vow to bring healing to as many beings as you can.

2. The Precept to Abstain from Taking What is Not Given

This precept is often translated as not stealing, but it goes beyond obvious theft to include not taking anything that is not given. If, say, you find an object lying on the ground, such as a ten-dollar bill, you can have it, but you must first make a genuine attempt to locate the rightful owner. In the healing arts, this precept expands to include not charging for healing that you are incapable of providing, and not making health care cost prohibitive.

3. The Precept to Abstain from Sexual Misconduct

This precept is actually about not committing adultery. Acts of sexual violence and molestation fall under the first precept of not harming. If you look at the Buddha's teachings as being primarily about having a harmonious life without suffering, you can see how adultery leads to a disharmonious life, not only for the couple but for the family and the village. This precept also includes not engaging in sex with someone who is under another person's care, or with minors. In the context of medical workers, it becomes the rule found in all medical traditions that doctors must refrain from sexual relations with patients.

4. The Precept to Abstain from False Speech

This precept is not simply about refraining from lying but also is inclusive of all speech that causes suffering, such as gossip, maligning others, and idle chatter. In a healing arts practice, it includes being honest about your medical skills and not speaking ill of other doctors in order to gain patients.

5. The Precept to Abstain from Intoxicants

There are several reasons for the precept against intoxication. One reason is that when one is intoxicated one is more likely to break the other precepts. A second is that experiences had while intoxicated are more clouded in illusion. A third is that because it is karmically very difficult to be born as a human being, using substances that hurt the body and cloud the mind is a wasted opportunity. For a medical worker, however, it takes on another reason: when you are intoxicated, you cannot reliably use your medical skills to help someone in need.

These five precepts are the ones that most Buddhists undertake. Monks hold many more precepts, with three additional ones of interest here, as these three extra precepts are often undertaken on certain days by lay people as well. You may wish to hold these precepts in addition to the five, on full and new moons, on holy days, or on your birthday. On these days the precept of sexual misconduct is changed to complete abstinence from sex and the following precepts are added:

The Precept to Abstain from Food After Midday

Monks abstain from eating after the midday meal every day, but many lay Buddhists will undertake this on special days. For monks there are exceptions, as they can eat certain foods, including dairy and chocolate. The reason for the exceptions is so that the monks do not become too depleted, especially in colder seasons, when some extra nourishment is needed. Lay people who are only occasionally holding the eight precepts may choose to forego all foods. Drinks, however, are allowed.

The Precept to Abstain from Frivolous Entertainment

This includes movies, books, music, dancing, and playing. On days when the eight precepts are held, one might instead read books on the dharma and sit in contemplation or meditation. This precept also includes not adorning the body with things like jewelry, perfume, or fancy clothes.

The Precept to Abstain from Sleeping in Luxurious or High Beds

This is about refraining from luxury in general on this day, and includes lounging in plush or tall chairs. It is about being simple and humble.

I have presented the precepts as they have been taught to me, without my personal interpretations or judgments about them. Of course, there is much variance in how they are interpreted. Some say that as long as you don't kill a being yourself, it is okay to eat meat, while others maintain that this is akin to hiring an assassin and then saying you are not responsible for the death they cause. Some say that adultery is any sex outside a marriage, while others say that it depends on the arrangement of that marriage; for example, if a couple agrees to be polyamorous, then there is room for sexual relations outside the marriage without breaking a precept. Some say that the precept of abstaining from intoxicants means that one should not become inebriated, while others interpret the meaning as not even a sip of wine is allowable. These are debates that linger in the Buddhist community. It should be remembered that these are vows one makes to oneself, so ultimately, you must look to your own heart for the interpretation.

When you make a vow, a precept, you make a promise to yourself. When you uphold this promise you are strengthened by it, but when you break this promise it weakens you. For this reason you should only make precepts that you intend to strive to keep. If, for example, you know that you like to get high on the weekends, and you have no intention of stopping, then it is not the time in your life to take the fifth precept. One does not have to be perfect to take precepts; in fact, if one was perfect there would be no need to take them at all. But one should actually be striving to uphold them. Also, the precepts are not rules. This is not a concept of sin and punishment. Precepts are simply things that are conducive to a harmonious life and the path toward enlightenment.

CHAPTER NINE

Taking Care

MEDICAL SCIENCES are imperative to any culture, and I have a deep love of the healing arts, but the most important aspect of healing may just be how we live our daily lives. Through understanding elemental constitution and imbalance, and by talking to people about their daily habits, you can learn to give guidance for self-care that will reach far beyond a weekly, monthly, or once-in-a-blue-moon visit to a health care provider. And so now we move into self-care—self-care for you, the medicine practitioner, and self-care for the community you care for.

Eight Daily Habits

General

Remember in the chapter on Disease and Imbalance, we learned about the Three Causes of Imbalance, and contained within the three causes was Daily Routine, or the Eight Daily Habits? There it was presented simply as how our daily routine leads to imbalance, because our daily habits are the primary cause of imbalance. Here, let's look at how our daily habits can help us to maintain good health.

1. *Eating Habits*
- Eat quality unprocessed foods.
- Whenever possible, eat organic, whole foods that are home cooked.
- Do not eat microwaved food. The biomedical debate about irradiated food aside, traditional doctors agree that microwaved food lacks essential vitality.
- Eat when you are hungry, not famished, and stop eating when you are satisfied, not full.
- Eat food that is well cooked and warm, whenever possible, as cold and uncooked foods are hard on the digestive fire.
- Eat seasonal fruits and vegetables.
- *In hot weather,* eat sweet, bitter, and astringent foods, and reduce consumption of pungent and sour foods.
- *In cold weather,* eat hot pungent (i.e. black pepper), sour, and astringent foods, and reduce salty and bitter foods.
- In rainy/windy weather, eat aromatic, warming foods (i.e. cinnamon and cumin), sweet and oily foods, and reduce consumption of astringent and bitter foods.
- Eat your last meal of the day before 7 p.m.

2. Postural Habits

- Try to spend approximately equal time throughout a twenty-four hour period lying down, sitting, and standing.
- Create as ergonomic a work environment as you can.
- Cultivate awareness of repetitive motion habits that may lead to physical imbalance.

3. Sleep Habits

Sleep is necessary to rejuvenate, and lack of sleep has a negative effect on digestion and the kidneys, which are associated with essence. Most people need four to eight hours of sleep, but only people who are very sedentary and meditate a lot can do well with closer to four hours. We are designed to get our best sleep between the hours of 10 p.m. and 5 a.m., waking during the Wind time, before sunrise. If you wake up after sunrise, then you are waking up during the lethargic Watery time, and you will not be as invigorated. Because children are in a naturally Watery time of life, busy building essence, they need to sleep more, so these rules do not apply until about age sixteen.

- Sleep six to eight hours per night.
- Wake within the last hour before sunrise.
- Do not sleep during the day (traditional medicine does not favor naps. I know!).
- Sleep on your side, with your head on a pillow.
- Avoid sleeping with a fan blowing on you, as it will distort your Wind.
- Go to sleep before 10 p.m., so that you fall asleep during the Water time of the evening. If you stay up past 10 p.m., it can become harder to fall asleep. Also, while the Fire time in the day, from 10 a.m. to 2 p.m., is a time when Fire digests food, the Fire time at night, between 10 p.m. and 2 a.m., is when Fire is involved in liver repair, which happens while you are sleeping.
- Since Wind element rises, anything that brings the energy down will assist with sleep. This might be a foot massage, soaking the feet, or rubbing oil on the feet.

4. Exercise Habits

- If possible, exercise during the Wind times of the day, in the early morning and the late afternoon.
- Intense cardiovascular exercise is not recommended in traditional medicine, as it is seen as being overly strenuous on the heart.
- If possible, find exercise that is enjoyable.
- Exercise must be separate from work. People who have physically demanding jobs still need to exercise, as most physically demanding work is depleting rather than nourishing. Healthy, enjoyable exercise, such as walking, bike riding, swimming, and so on, may be tiring, but it nourishes us rather than depleting us.

5. Work Habits

- Whenever possible, avoid overworking.
- Avoid jobs that require working at night. People who work at night and sleep in the

day inevitably develop Wind imbalances, which can then lead to further elemental imbalances.

- If you must work at night, try to follow the elemental times. Fall asleep during Water hours (after sunrise), eat during Fire hours (middle of the night), and awaken during Wind hours (in the late afternoon).
- Avoid jobs that deal in weapons, abuse humans, involve killing other beings, or the sale of intoxicants and poisons, or any other job that feels ethically or spiritually wrong to you.

6. Temperature

Keep your home, work environment, and car as close to the natural temperature as you can, while keeping it cool or warm enough that you don't tax your body or create suffering. So if you need to cool things down a bit because your environment is in a heat extreme you can, but don't run the air conditioner in such a manner that you walk from outside heat into refrigerator cold.

7. Natural Urges

- Do not suppress the urge to sneeze, defecate, urinate, pass gas, yawn, or burp.
- Breathe fully, exhaling fully to eliminate Wind waste product.
- Engage in moderate, healthy, and consensual sexual activity.

8. Emotional Habits

As much as possible, avoid engaging in extremes of emotions. It is natural to feel happiness and sadness in life, but when we spend too much time in the extremes of emotion, such as depression, rage, and giddiness, we cause elemental imbalances. To learn to cultivate balanced emotions, focus on the *Brahmavihara* of equanimity and practice meditation. Sometimes, the idea of avoiding excessive pleasure is confusing for people. The problem is that pleasure is short-lived, and worry about losing it causes suffering.

Daily Habits: Specific Elements

The above recommendations are generalized. What follows is advice for when specific elements are dominating. In general, this would apply to your core elemental constitution; however, if an imbalance has led to a different element dominating in the moment, follow the advice for that element.

1. Wind

- Try to stick to schedules. Go to bed at the same time each night, awake at the same time, and eat at specified times.
- Apply oil to your body daily. Raw sesame oil is preferable.
- Eat highly nutritious foods with aromatic spices.
- Eat many small meals throughout the day instead of three large meals.
- Avoid raw foods, especially at night. Also, be aware that Wind element, once excited,

likes to further agitate itself by engaging in food extremes such as fasting, raw food diets, and other strong dietary restrictions. At first this will feel good to Windy people, but eventually it will only further the imbalance. Raw foods are particularly bad for Wind and Water.

- Eat oily, nutritious foods, such as healthy fats and oils; quality dairy products, if you eat dairy; and nuts.
- Eat steamed, well-cooked foods that are easily digested.
- Do not sleep during the day.
- Try to go to bed at night when you first feel tired. If you stay up past the first wave of exhaustion, insomnia is likely.
- Try to sleep eight hours per night.
- Do breathing exercises to balance the Winds.
- Do not work or study too much without movement breaks.
- Do not engage in excessive sexual activity.
- Meditate. Of course, this is recommended for everyone, but for Windy people it is essential.
- Engage in grounded physicality such as gardening—things that put you firmly in your body and working with the earth.

2. Fire

- Reduce consumption of spicy foods.
- Eat regular large meals rather than snacking throughout the day.
- Fiery people can generally eat most foods so long as their digestive fire is strong.
- Be careful of overbalancing through use of too many cooling foods, but do lean toward them.
- Moderate sexual activity is healthy for Fiery people.
- Sleep seven to eight hours of sleep per night.
- Go to sleep before midnight.
- Exercise moderately. If possible when the surroundings are cool and out of the sun.
- Coffee[76] in moderation is okay, but it's better for Fiery people if they put some cream (including nut milks) and a healthy sweetener in it.
- Avoid drugs[77] and alcohol. Of course, everyone should be wary of these substances, but they can be extra hard on Fire.
- Eat something bitter every day, such as arugula, radicchio, and mustard greens.

---

76 Coffee is cooling, bitter. It stimulates Wind, but in a fairly reasonable way when ingested in moderation, but is not good for those with excited Wind. It helps with diarrhea that stems from lack of Wind. Adding sweeteners and milk is good for Fire constitution people, and ill effects on the stomach can be mitigated by adding cardamom, cinnamon, and nutmeg. Coffee is number one a heart stimulant.

77 Marijuana depletes your Fire, makes the Fire useless, depletes the essence, and creates dryness in the body. Use nurturing therapies like coconut oils (ingested); even though the body will be cool inside, there is so much dryness the coconut oil will help.

3. Water

- Avoid coffee
- In the morning, avoid cold foods such as fruit, yogurt, smoothies, and so on. Reduce consumption of cold and raw foods.
- In the morning, eat hot cereal, eggs, toast, and so on.
- Avoid eating raw foods. Raw foods are particularly bad for Water and Wind. If eating raw or cooling foods, only do so at midday.
- Low to no consumption of meat, and low consumption of sweet foods.
- Eat cooked vegetables, rice, and pungent spices.
- Eat very light dinners, or skip dinner.
- Wake early and do not sleep during the day.
- Avoid oversleeping. Ideally, sleep six to seven hours between 10 p.m. and 7 a.m.
- Engage in active exercise with lots of movement.
- Healthy sexual activity is beneficial for Watery people.
- Drink two glasses of hot water with lemon or lime juice, honey, and black pepper every morning before meals.

Common Ailments and Thai Medicine

This section looks at a small sample of common ailments through the Thai medicine lens. Because traditional medicine is tailored to the individual rather than a pathology label, ultimately one must understand the theory and spend time with the ailing person. I have sought to choose some examples of maladies that allow for a generic answer, but the individual, their age, the season, all of the factors from the imbalance causation lists should be considered in actual application.

Acute Injuries

Common acute injuries are sprains and strains, contusions, broken bones, and various forms of tissue damage. Generally, acute injuries are bled by puncturing the wounded area with a needle and then applying a cup to draw out the blood. This is done a few times in the first few days. If the skin is broken, apply the Thai Healing Salve found on page 143. If the injury has inflammation and swelling, it also needs to be cooled. In Thai medicine, cooling is accomplished either by using herbs that have cooling properties, or simply by applying a cool cloth that has been dipped in cool water. The cloth will have to be repeatedly dipped in the water as the body will heat it quickly.

Traditional medicine across Asia does not ice acute injuries. While Western medicine is quite fond of icing acute injuries, traditional medicine holds that ice causes short-term relief but brings long-term damage. That ankle that just never quite fully healed after being sprained? That old knee injury that acts up every time the temperature drops? These kinds of ongoing injuries are frequently attributed to icing during the acute phase. In Tom Bisio's brilliant book *A Tooth From a Tiger's Mouth: How to Treat Your Injuries with Powerful Healing Secrets of the Great Chinese Warriors* he writes:

Ice is very useful for preserving things in a static state. It slows or halts the decay of food and dead bodies but does not help damaged tissue repair itself.

Ice does reduce the initial swelling and inflammation of a fresh injury, and it does reduce pain, but at a cost. Contracting local blood vessels and tissues by freezing them inhibits the restoration of normal circulation. The static blood and fluids congeal, contract, and harden with icing, making them harder or impossible to disperse later. It is not uncommon to see a sprained ankle that was iced still slightly swollen more than a year after the original injury... Icing an injured area causes further contraction in muscles, ligaments, and tendons that are already contracted in reaction to being overstretched. This further slows the healing process and prevents the return of normal movement.

Since learning about how traditional medicine views icing I have paid close attention to the subject. I have found that, almost without fail, the people I meet who have injuries that will not fully heal iced them heavily at some point.

Anxiety

Anxiety comes from Wind and Fire. Fire is a primary element of emotions, and it distorts the Wind. Liver troubles can also create anxiety because the liver is the primary organ of Fire. Earth and Water elements are needed. Massage is beneficial, as it brings people back in touch with their bodies, which are Earth. Massage oils into the body, and follow the protocols for anxiety presented in the physical therapies chapter. If what is manifesting is fear rather than anxiety, then it is more likely a Water issue, as fear is related to not knowing. If what is manifesting is worry it is likely an Earth association, as worry is fear that comes from caring.

Bloating

There are two kinds of bloating: bloating from Water and bloating from gas. Bloating from gas is caused by excessive Wind, which is caused by deficient Fire. The digestive fire isn't processing the food, so it ferments and creates gas. Bloating from Water happens when there is a Fire deficiency as well, but in this case there is also deficient Wind, as the Water should be moving out through the skin and such but is instead just sitting in the tissue. If there is Wind in the stomach that needs to be released, eat a tiny pinch of real camphor. This will make you burp immediately. Real camphor is an off-white, ever so slightly brownish color, so if your camphor is pure white, it is synthetic.

Bronchitis

Excess Water, deficient Wind. The lungs need to be dried out. Dry saunas can be beneficial. For mucous, you can burn or steam pine wood.

Candida

Excess Water, deficient Fire. Look to diet and daily habits to nourish the Fire element and calm the Water element. Reduce intake of cold, heavy, sweet, and sticky foods, while increasing intake of warming foods.

Canker Sores

Canker sores are generally a sign of too much internal heat or toxins in the digestive system. They are not related to the herpes virus. If they appear on their own they are likely from heat, but if they result from mouth wounds, then they are likely from toxins. Watermelon frost, which can be purchased from Asian food markets in the medicinal section, may help bring relief, but to stop the occurrence, either Fire-balancing herbs and diet and lifestyle changes must be adopted; if it is from toxins, then detoxification with the guidance of a healing arts professional is recommended. This said, traditional medicine aside for a moment, using toothpaste that doesn't contain any sodium lauryl sulphate can reduce canker sore occurrence by amazing amounts.

Colicky Babies

Usually something is bothering them that you might not be aware of. Clean their space, make sure there is fresh air, massage coconut oil into their skin. This kind of colic is often seen at dusk and dawn, the windy times of day when spirits and such are more readily felt. Colic can also be troubles with the gross Winds causing pain in the abdomen, in which case a little hing (asofeotida) and tulsi mixed with the baby's milk can be beneficial.

Constipation

Constipation can come from a lack of Water (hard stools) or an excess of Water (sticky stools). It can also come from slack Wind element (normal stools that just don't move easily). If the Wind is not moving, give a purgative such as senna, but be careful as this will cause cramping that can be painful. This can be mitigated by also giving aromatic herbs like cardamom and young (not too hot) ginger. If there is too much Water, turmeric can be beneficial, and if there is not enough water, hydrate.

Diarrhea

Diarrhea can come from excited Wind element moving things along too quickly (there will be undigested food in the stools), or it can come from excited Water element (very wet feces). If the diarrhea is caused by Wind element, eat bulky and somewhat oily foods, such as potatoes cooked with oil. If the diarrhea is caused by Water, eat astringent things such as turmeric, pomegranate peel, or mangosteen peel. You can also make a tea from powdered unroasted coffee beans and drink it.

Ear Infections

Squeeze a little garlic juice into ear.

Essence Depletion

We are born with strong essence, which gives us energy throughout childhood and life. Essence is related to sexual organs and the kidneys and is supported by good sleep, nutritious food, clean water, healthy exercise, and nourishing, moderate sexual activity. (I suspect that homemade cookies help, as well.) Many things cause essence depletion, so if someone is haggard, washed out, and lacking in vitality, you first need to figure out what might be causing it. Drugs, alcohol, and lack of sleep are all very common causes, as is eating unnutritious foods or having poor digestive fire, such that you are not absorbing nutrients.

Depleted Water element is also connected to depleted essence. Women who are on their menses experience temporary essence depletion and need to nourish their essence at this time, and men who ejaculate frequently will deplete essence as well. Treat depleted essence with raw cow's milk or fresh homemade almond milk,[78] cashews, cardamom, saffron, and dates. Make sure that they are hydrated with quality water or coconut water, and take blood tonics such as safflower and/or cinnamon tea, angelica root, or blackstrap molasses.

Eczema

Rub coconut oil into the skin. The healing salve formula on page 143 is also very good for eczema.

Fibromyalgia

Fibromyalgia can benefit significantly from the use of Wind liniment and hot herbal compresses. You can use the common warming compresses. Be cautious of common Thai massage routines as while they may feel good while being applied, they frequently cause pain flareups in the ensuing days. Just stick with complete hot compress sessions until the patient begins to recover and is able to tolerate stronger work.

Heartburn

Heartburn indicates a problem with ascending Wind. Most likely ascending Wind is being distorted by excessive Fire in the digestive tract. Eat cooling, gentle foods such as yogurt and rice soup. Chew dried calamus root, or make a tea out of it, and work the ascending Wind point.

Insomnia

Insomnia results from excess Wind, and usually a deficiency in Water. The Water isn't there to smooth the Wind out. It could also come from excess Fire exciting the Wind. Either way you need to increase the Water in the body, both in the tissue and in the emotional body. Eating sour foods is good (they are warm but increase Water) also bitter and salty foods. Soak, swim, or bathe in warm water that isn't extremely hot. Use warm herbal compresses, and massage oil into the body. Before bed, pull the energy downwards by soaking the feet in warm water or massaging oil into the feet. Also, those with insomnia should try to go to sleep when the first wave of tiredness hits them at night.

Joint Pain

Gentle traction on the joints, massage liniments for the joints into the area, and eat mung beans boiled with ginger and jaggery or any natural sugar. Pain is Wind. Even if there is inflammation, Wind is involved. The Wind can be excessive or deranged. Joints are a place of Wind, as joints

---

78 The pre-packaged almond milk found in stores has very little actual almond milk in it, being primarily made of water and thickeners. Real almond milk is thick and creamy on its own, and does not require thickening agents. In traditional medicine, raw almond milk is considered to be the nondairy substance that most closely resembles mammal milk.

are places in the body where Wind gets stuck. Joints are a big problem for Wind. This is why bone setting is used, as a means to release the trapped Wind in the joints. Cracking your joints too much can distort Wind, though, so the best way to release the Wind in the joints is through gentle traction of the joints. If joint pain is caused by overgrowth of bone or compaction of the joints, then this is an Earth problem.

Menstruation

Do extensive bodywork on the legs, including massaging liniment into the trenches, and use hot herbal compresses on the stomach and low back. Eat warming foods and foods that build blood, such as greens, sea vegetables, foods cooked in cast iron pots, and blackstrap molasses. In general, coconut water is beneficial for female hormones, but it is too cool for drinking during menstruation.

Overheating/Heatstroke

Eat watermelon, and rub the white inner rind on your skin. Scrape the top of the head, and any other area that has been beaten by the sun.

Restless Leg Syndrome

Do blood stops, massage with Wind liniment, and eat healthy oils. Do exercises that exhaust the legs, and drink tonic water for the quinine. Restless leg syndrome is a Wind imbalance, so all things that balance Wind should be helpful.

Sciatica

With sciatica, Earth is affecting Wind in the form of either muscles or bone impacting the nerve. Only external bodywork therapies can help. If sciatica is coming from the lumbar spine, use techniques that open the lumbar spine, and apply hot herbal compresses. Massage nerve liniment or St. John's wort oil into the laminal groove, and work the legs. If the sciatica comes from the piriformis muscle pressing on the sciatic nerve, massage the gluteal area, do tok sen if trained, and use contract-relax techniques if so trained.

Spinal Pain

When compression of vertebrae and degeneration in the spine and vertebral discs causes pain, you can massage oil infused with St. John's wort and calamus or the Wind liniment into the laminal groove on the side of the spine. Eat oily nutritious foods such as nuts, and traction the spine for sustained periods. Hot herbal compress massage can help to relieve the surrounding tissue tension. Inversion tables can also be useful to bring space to the spine.

Vaginal Yeast Infections

Wrap a clove of garlic in cheesecloth, and tie with a string. Leave the string for a long tail to remove with, and insert the garlic inside the vagina. Leave in for several hours.

Bibliography

Bamber, Scott (1987). "Illness Taxonomy on Traditional Thai Medicine." In *Proceedings of the 3rd International Conference on Thai Studies.* Vol. 3, Part 2. Canberra: Australian National University, pp. 605–613.

Bamber, Scott (1982). "Lom: An Examination of a Term Used in Association with Illness in Traditional Thai Medicine." BA (Asian Studies) Honors subthesis. Canberra: Australian National University.

Bamber, Scott (1989). "Trope and Taxonomy: An Examination of the Classification and Treatment of Illness in Traditional Thai Medicine." PhD thesis, Canberra: Australian National University.

Beyer, C. (1907). "About Siamese Medicine." In *Journal of the Siam Society.* Vol. 4.

Bharabhutanonda, Vilaiporn (1980). "The Medical Role of the 'Doctor Bhikku' in Bangkok and Rural Communities." In *Journal of National Research Council of Thailand.* Vol. 12, pp. 11–60.

Birla, Ghanshyam Singh (2007). *Introduction to Hast Jyotish: Ancient Eastern System of Palmistry.* Chénéville, Canada: Galaxy Publications & Recordings.

Bisio, Tom (2004). *A Tooth From The Tiger's Mouth: How to Treat Your Injuries with Powerful Healing Secrets of the Great Chinese Warriors.* New York: Fireside Books.

Bradley, D. B. (1967). "Siamese Theory and Practice of Medicine." Bangkok Calendar 1865. Reprinted in *Social Science Review.* Vol. 5/2, Bangkok, Thailand. pp. 103–119.

Brun, Viggo and Trond Schumacher (1987). *Traditional Herbal Medicine in Northern Thailand: With a List of Plants.* Berkeley: University of California Press.

Bunratanakoonkit, Latdawan and Thanoomchit Suphaawitaa (1975). *Chüü phüüt samunphrai lä prajoot. (Names of Medicinal Plants and Their Use).* Bangkok, Thailand.

Bunsri, Kasem (1973). "Praphenii suu khwan." In *Watthanatham Thai.* Vol. 13 / 8, pp. 12–15.

Chaichakan, Sinthoon (1977). *Khuumüü süksaa lakwichaa pheesatchakam phään booraan. (A Study Manual in the Principles of Traditional Pharmacy).* Chiang Mai, Thailand: The Traditional Clinic in Northern Thailand.

Chanthawimon, Samai (1954). "Kaanphäät khoong pratheet thai: rachakaan thii saam – rachakaan thii sii (Medicine in Thailand: The 3rd and the 4th Reigns)." In *Journal of the Medical Association of Thailand.* Vol. 37, pp. 317–330.

Chenxia, Wang (1996). *Palmar Lines: Chinese Palmistry in Medical Application.* Jinan, China: Shandong Friendship.

Davis, Richard (1974). "Muang Metaphysics: A Study of Northern Thai Myth and Ritual." PhD thesis. Sydney, Australia: University of Sydney.

Diamond, Jared (1997). *Guns, Germs, and Steel: The Fates of Human Societies.* Norton & Company, Inc.: New York.

Domett, Kathryn M. (2001). *Health in Late Prehistoric Thailand.* Oxford, UK: British Archaeological Reports Series.

Egawa, Janey and Nathaniel Tashima (1982). *Indigenous Healers in Southeast Asian Refugee Communities.* San Francisco, CA: Pacific Asian Mental Health Research Project.

Farnsworth, Norman R. (ed.) (1992). *Thai Medicinal Plants: Recommended for Primary Health Care System.* Bangkok, Thailand: Medicinal Plant Information Center.

Forbes, Andrew & Henley, David (1997). *Khon Muang: People and Principalities of North Thailand.* Chiang Mai, Thailand: Asia Film House.

Gerhards, Paul (2007). *Mapping the Dharma: A Concise Guide to the Middle Way of the Buddha.* Vancouver, BC: Parami Press.

Green, James (2000). *The Herbal Medicine-Maker's Handbook: A Home Manual.* Berkeley, CA: The Crossing Press (a division of Ten Speed Press).

Halpern, Joel M. (1963). "Traditional Medicine and the Role of the Phi in Laos." In *Eastern Anthropologist.* Vol. 16, pp. 191–200.

Heinze, Ruth-Inge (1977). "Nature and Function of Some Therapeutic Techniques in Thailand." In *Asian Folklore Studies.* Vol. 37 / 2, pp. 85–104.

Heinze, Ruth-Inge (1982). *Tham Khwan: How to Contain the Essence of Life. A Socio-Psychological Comparison of A Thai Custom.* Kent Ridge: Singapore University Press.

Heinze, Ruth-Inge (1971). "The Khwan: A Test Case for the Syncretic Pattern of Thai Buddhism." MA thesis, Asian Studies. Berkeley: University of California.

Heinze, Ruth-Inge (1988). *Trance and Healing in Southeast Asia Today.* Bangkok, Thailand: White Lotus Press.

Hofbauer, R. (1943). "A Medical Retrospect of Thailand." In *Journal of the Thailand Research Society.* Vol. 34, pp. 183–200.

Hoskin, John and Jean-Léo Dugast (1993). *The Supernatural in Thai Life.* Bangkok, Thailand: Tamarind Press.

Ionescu-Tongyonk, J. (1981). "Explication of Wind Illness in Nothern Thailand." In *Transcultural Psychiatric Research Review.* Vol. 18, pp. 42–45.

Janthagul, Suddinand (1994). *The Sacred Book of Buddhist Chants: Pali - Thai - English Translation.* Bangkok, Thailand: Thammasapa.

Jaspan, M. A. (1969). *Traditional Medical Theory in South-East Asia.* Hull, UK: University of Hull.

Johaari, Harish (1990). *Numerology with Tantra, Ayurveda, and Astrology: A Key to Human Behavior.* Rochester, VT: Destiny Books.

Kacera, Walter 'Shantree' (2006). *Ayurvedic Tongue Diagnosis.* Twin Lakes, WI: Lotus Press.

Khanitthanan, Wilaiwan (1988). "Khamriak Khwan: Banthük Prawatsaat Booraan Lä Sanyalak Lä Khwaam Maai (Calling the Khwan: Notes on the History, Characteristics, and Meaning)." In *Ruam bot khwaam prawatsaat.* Vol. 10, pp. 114–124.

Khunphakdii, Nanthana (1987). *Kaanwikhro Khwaam Chüa Khoong Chaai Thai Nai Sawattiraksaa.* (*A Study on the Beliefs of Thai Men Concerning Healthcare*). Bangkok, Thailand: Silapakorn University, BE 2530.

Lagan, Heather Alicia (2011). *Chaldean Numerology For Beginners: How Your Name & Birthday Reveal Your True Nature & Life Plan.* Woodbury, MN: Llewellyn Publications.

Lampang Health Development Project (1978). *A Thai Primary Health Care Approach.* Bangkok, Thailand: Ministry of Public Health.

Lüangkääsoon, Prasööt (1962). "Prawat Kaanphäät Nai Samai Lang Khoong Ratchakaan Thii Haa (The Medical History of the Latter Part of the Fifth Reign [1889-1910])." In *Siriraj Journal,* pp. 562–567.

Maguire, Jack (2001). *Essential Buddhism: A Complete Guide to Beliefs and Practices.* New York: Pocket Books, a division of Simon & Schuster Inc.

Mettanando, Bhikkhu: (1998). "Meditation and Healing in the Theravada Buddhist Order of Thailand and Laos." PhD thesis, Hamburg, Germany: University of Hamburg.

Mills, M. B. (1995). "Attack of the Widow Ghosts: Gender, Death, and Modernity in Northeast Thailand." In *Bewitching Women, Pious Men: Gender and Body Polities in Southeast Asia.* Edited by A. Ong and M.G.

Peletz. Berkeley: University of California Press.

Muecke, Marjorie A. (1979). "An Explication of 'Wind Illness' in Northern Thailand." In *Culture, Medicine and Psychiatry*. Vol. 3, pp. 267-300.

Mulholland, Jean (1979). "Thai Traditional Medicine: Ancient Thought and Practice in a Thai Context." In *Journal of the Siam Society*. Vol. 67 / 2, pp. 80-115.

Mulholland, Jean (1987). "Medicine, Magic and Evil Spirits: Study of a Text on Thai Traditional Paediatrics." *In Faculty of Asian Studies Monographs: New Series No. 8.* Canberra: Australian National University.

Mulholland, Jean (1989). "Herbal Medicine in Paediatrics. Translation of a Thai Book of Genesis." In *Faculty of Asian Studies Monographs, New Series No. 14.* Canberra: Australian National University.

Nidtheet, Sukkhit (Khun) (1973). *Aaayuraweet Süksaa: Wichaaphäät Hään Booraan (Ayurvedic Studies: Traditional Medicine)*. 2nd ed. Bangkok, Thailand.

Nimmanahaeminda, Prakong (1978). *Khwan Lä Khamriak Khwan (Khwan and Calling the Khwan)*. Bangkok, Thailand: Laannaa Thai Khadii, pp. 106-136.

Phäätsaat Songkhro (Medical Assistance) (1964-1976). 3 vols. Bangkok, Thailand: Society of the School of Traditional Medicine, Wat Pho.

Phatthanaa, Phichaan (1966). *Khwaampenmaa Khoong Kaanphäät Müang Thai (Accounts from the History of Medicine in Thailand)*. Bangkok, Thailand.

Phinthoong, Prichaa (1987). "Kaan suu khwan (Calling the Khwan)." In *Prapheenii Thai booraan Isaan*. Ubol-Rajathani, Thailand, pp. 246-297.

Phinthoon, Prichaa (1987). "Kaan too aayu (Expenditure of Life)." In *Prapheenii Thai booraan Isaan*. Ubol-Rajathani, Thailand, pp. 2-56.

Phitsanuprasaatwet, Phrayaa (1970). *Weetchasüksaa Phäätsaat Sangkheep (Medical Studies: An Outline)*. Bangkok, Thailand: Roongrian Weedchasamoosoon.

Phitsanuprasaatwet, Phrayaa (ed.) (1909). *Weetchasüksaa Phäätthayasaat Sangkheep (Manual for Students of Traditional Medicine)*. 3 Vols., 2nd ed. Bangkok, Thailand.

Photchananukrom phäät pheesaat thai (A Dictionary of the Thai Medical and Pharmaceutical Terms) (1964). Bangkok, Thailand: The Ayurvedic Society of Bangkok.

Photchanaanukrom Phäät Pheesat Thai: Chabap Maattrathaan (Dictionary of Thai Medicine and Pharmacy: Standard Edition) (1964). Bangkok, Thailand: Association of Traditional Pharmacy and Ayurvedic Medicine of Thailand.

Photchanaanukrom Sap Phäät Angkrit-Thai Chabap Raatchabanthitayasathaan (English-Thai Medical Dictionary of the Royal Institute) (1965). Bangkok, Thailand: Royal Institute.

Phrommanee, Prasoet and Parinyaa Uthitchalaanon (eds.) (1973). *Tamraa Pheesatchakam Thai Phään Booraan (Textbook of Thai Traditional Pharmacy)*. Bangkok, Thailand: College of Traditional Medicine, Wat Mahathat.

Phuvanatnaranubala, Thirachai & Kornaek Khongpurttiroj (2010). *Know Your Future: Thai Astrology A Step By Step Guide*. Roply, Hants, UK: O Books, an imprint of John Hunt Publishing.

Poulsen, Anders (2008). *Childbirth and Tradition in Northeast Thailand: 40 Years of Development and Cultural Change*. Copenhagen, Denmark: NIAS Press.

Pramuan Saphakhun *Yaa Thai Waaduai Phrüksaachaat Watthuthaat Lä Satwatthu Naanaachanit (A Compilation of the Properties of Various Thai Drugs from the Botanical, Mineral, and Animal Kingdoms)* (1963-1969). 3 vols. Bangkok, Thailand: The Society of the School of Traditional Medicine in Thailand, Wat Pho.

Rajadhon, Phya Anuman (1962). "The Khwan and its Ceremonies." In *Journal of the Siam Society*. Vol. 50/2, pp. 119-164.

Rajadhon, Phya Anuman (1969). *Essay on Thai Folklore.* Bangkok, Thailand: Editions Duang Kamol.

Ratarasaan, Somchintana Thongthäo (1986). *The Principles and Concept of Thai Classical Medicine.* PhD thesis, University of Wisconsin-Madison.

Rüangsuwan, Charubut (1981). "Kham Suu Khwan (Texts for Calling the Khwan)." In *Watthanatham Thai.* Vol. 20/7, pp. 44–55.

Salguero, Pierce (2007). *Traditional Thai Medicine: Buddhism, Animism, Ayurveda.* Prescott, AZ: Hohm Press.

Saralamp, Promjit, et al. (1996). *Medicinal Plants in Thailand. Vol I.* Bangkok, Thailand: Amarin Printing and Publishing.

Saralamp, Promjit, et al. (1997). *Medicinal Plants in Thailand. Vol II.* Bangkok, Thailand: Chulalongkorn University Boo.

Society of the School of Traditional Medicine in Thailand, Wat Pho (1969). *Khuumüü Kaansüksaa Wichaa Phääsaatchakoon Thai (A Manual for Studies in Thai Pharmacy).* Bangkok, Thailand.

Society of the School of Traditional Medicine in Thailand, Wat Pho (1970).

Khuumüü Kaansüksaa Wichaa Weetchakam. (*A Manual for Medical Studies*). Bankok, Thailand.

Somchintana, Ratarsarn (1986). *The Principles and Concepts of Thai Classical Medicine.* Bangkok, Thailand: Thai Khadi Research Institute, Thammasat University.

Soonlam, Seek. *Näo Khwaamruu Kaansüksaa Weetchakam Phään Booraan (Insights in the Study of Traditional Medicine).* Bangkok, Thailand: Society of Traditional Doctors, Wat Mahathat. No date.

Mahidol University, Faculty of Pharmacy (1986). *Specification of Thai Medicinal Plants, Vol. 1: A Guide to the Identification and Authentication of Some Thai Medicinal Plants.* Bangkok, Thailand.

Tambiah, Stanley J. (1970). *Buddhism and the Spirit Cults in North-East Thailand.* Cambridge, UK: Cambridge University Press.

Tamraa Jaa Chaarük Wat Raacha-oorot Lä Phra-oosot Phra Naaraai (Medical Manuals: Inscriptions at Raja-orot Temple and the Medicines of Narai) (1997). Bangkok, Thailand: Ministry of Education.

Tamraa Pheesatchakam Thai Phään Booraan (A Textbook in Traditional Thai Pharmacy) (1973). Bangkok, Thailand: Society of Traditional Doctors, Wat Mahathat.

Tamraa Pheesat Phrabaat Sondet Phranangklao Chaojuuhua (Medical Texts Which His Majesty King Rama III Had Engraved at Phra Chetuphon Temple [Wat Pho] in B.E.2375 [A.D. 1832]) (1977). Bangkok, Thailand: Association of the Traditional Medical School.

Tamraa Pramuan Lak Pheesat (A Textbook in the Fundamentals of Pharmacy) (1978). Bangkok, Thailand: School of Traditional Medicine, Wat Pho.

Tamraa Jaa Samunphrai Laannaa (Traditional Lanna Thai Medical Text) (1979). Compiled by Palm Leaf Text Studies Program. Chiang Mai, Thailand: Faculty of Social Sciences, University of Chiang Mai.

Terwiel, B.J. (1994). *Monks and Magic: An Analysis of Religious Ceremonies in Central Thailand.* Bangkok, Thailand: White Lotus Co., Ltd.

Uthidchalaanon, Pariyaa (1974). *Khampanyaai Wichaaphäät Phään Booraan (Explanations to Traditional Medicine).* Bangkok, Thailand: Traditional Doctor Study Division, Wat Mahathad.

Verma, Vinod (2013). *Numerology Based On Vedic Tradition.* Dunda Uttarakhand: Gayatri Book International.

Wongphaa, Samran (1952). "Prawat Kaanphäät Thai: Tamraayaa Chaak Silaachaarük Wat Raatcha-Oorasaaraam (History of Thai Medicine: The Medical Treatise Inscribed at Raja-Orasaram Temple)." In *Siriraj Journal,* Jan. 1952.

Zong, Xiao-Fan & Gary Liscum (1999). *Chinese Medical Palmistry: Your Health in Your Hand.* Boulder, CO: Blue Poppy Press.

APPENDIX A

Glossary of Thai and Pali Words

Aa-gàat - อากาศ - Air

Aa-gàat tâat - อากาศธาตุ - Space element

Aa-yú-sa mút-tăan - อายุสมุฏฐาน - Age Causative Factor

A-dtù-sa mút-tăan- อุตุสมุฏฐาน - Seasonal Causative Factor

A-pát-tá-bpìt-dtà - อพัทธะปิตตะ - Unbound Fire

Bpan-jà in-see - ปัญจอินทรีย์ - Five Sense Diagnosis

Bprà-dtoo lom - ประตูลม - Wind gate

Bprà-tâyt-sa mút-tăan - ประเทศสมุฏฐาน - Region/Climate

Bpìt-dtà - ปิตตะ - Fire. Stems from the Pāli word, pitta

Borapet - บอระเพ็ด - Thai herb. Tinospora cordifolia, also known as Guduchi.

Châat - ชาติ First stage on of imbalance

Cha phluu - ช้าพลู - Thai herb. Piper chaba. Also known as Wild Betel Leaf.

Dee bplee- ดีปลี - Thai herb. Piper longum. Also known as Long Pepper.

Dtaèk - แตก - Broken

Dtap awn - ตับอ่อน - Pancreas

Dtee - ตี - Beating

Gaala-sa mút-tăan - กาลสมุฏฐาน - Time Causative Factor

Gam-dao - กำเดา - Body heat

Gam rêrp - กำเริบ - Excited, Agitated, Amplified, Excessive

Gà-rì-sà - กรีส - Old Food

Gòt jùt - กดจุด - Release Points

Hăai bpai - หายไป - Disappeared, Lost, Missing

Hà-tai Wâata - หทัยวาต -Heart Wind

Hà-tai wát-tù - หทัยวัตถุ - Heart Hà-tai means heart, and components, things, or pieces.

Jàp chêep-pá-jon - จับชีพจร - Pulse Diagnosis

Jàláná - จะละนะ - Second stage two of imbalance

Jàyt moon plerng - เจตมูลเพลิง - Thai herb. Plumbago spp. Also known as Chitrak or Plumbago.

Jìt jai - จิตใจ - Heart mind

Karunā - Compassion

Khing - ขิง - Thai herb. Zingiber officinale. Ginger

Kon Muang - คนเมือง - town people

Kon song - คนทรงเจ้า - Medium (someone who channels unseen beings)

Kuut Săym-hà - คูธเสมหะ - Mucus of the Bowels

Kwăn - ขวัญ - Spirit of component body parts

Kwăn hăai - ขวัญหาย - Loss of kwăn

Lâyk sàat - เลขศาสตร์ - Numerology, or math

Lêuat - เลือด - Blood

Loh-hìt - โลหิต - Blood (medical terminology)

Lôok bprà-kóp - ลูกประคบ - Herbal compress

Maha Săn ni-bàat - มหาสันนิบาต - When all four elements are imbalanced

Mettā - Loving kindness

Mŏr meuang - หมอเมือง - Lanna doctor

Mŏr pĕe - หมอผี - Spirit Doctor

Muay Thai - มวยไทย - Thai kick boxing

Muditā - sympathetic joy

Pâet păen-boh-raan - แพทย์แผนโบราณ - Traditional Medicine

Pâet péun bâan khawng laan-naa - แพทย์พื้นบ้านของลานนา - Local Medicine of Lanna

Pâet păen tai - แพทย์แผนไทย - Thai medicine

Pâet péun bâan - แพทย์พื้นบ้าน - Local medicine

Pát-tá-bpìt-dtà - พัทธะปิตตะ - Bound or contained Fire

Pí-gaan - พิการ - Distorted, Deranged

Pinná - ภินนะ - Third stage three of imbalance

Pí-tee baai sĕe sòo kwăn พิธีบายศรีสู่ขวัญ Ceremony of reinforcing the kwăn.

Prá sŏng - พระสงฆ์ - Monk

Rang sŏng - ร่างทรง - Medium (someone who channels unseen beings)

Reeak kwan - เรียกขวัญ - A ceremony that calls the kwăn back

Reu-sĕe - ฤษี - Ascetic

Reu-sĕe dàt dton - ฤษีดัดตน Thai self care system

Rót bprîeow - รสเปรี้ยว - Sour

Rót fàat - รสฝาด - Astringent

Rót hŏm yen - รสหอมเย็น - Fragrant/Cool

Rót jèut - รสจืด - Tasteless

Rót kem - รสเค็ม - Salty

Rót kŏm - รสขม - Bitter

Rót man - รสมัน - Oily

Rót mao bèua - รสเมาเบื่อ - Toxic

Rót pèt rón - รสเผ็ดร้อน - Spicy/hot

Rót wăan - รสหวาน - Sweet

Sàat hàeng gaan doo laai meu - ศาสตร์แห่งการดูลายมือ - Palmistry

Sakhan - สะค้าน - Thai herb. Piper interruptum.

Saksit - ศักดิ์สิทธิ์ - Sacred

Sà-mùt-tăan aa-bpoh pí-gàt สมุฏฐานอาโปพิกัต - Water Causative Factor

Sà-mùt-tăan bpà-tà-wĕe tâat pí-gàt สมุฏฐานปถวีธาตุพิกัต - Earth Causative Factor

Sà-mùt-tăan dtay-choh-tâat pí-gàt - สมุฏฐานเตโชธาตุพิกัต - Fire Causative Factor

Sà-mùt-tăan waa-yoh-tâat pí-gàt - สมุฏฐานวาโยธาตุพิกัต - Wind causative factor

Săn ni-bàat - สันนิบาต - Multiple elements disturbed

Sat-ta-haka Wâata - สัตตะกะวาต - Knife Like Wind

Săym-hà -เสมหะ- Water. Stems from the Pāli word semha

Sên - เส้น - Many meanings, in this context, pathway of movement in the body

Som-dun - สมดุล - Balance, healthy, normal

Sŏr Săym-hà - ศอเสมหะ - Mucus of the Neck and Head

Sù-kŭm สุขุม - Temperature that is neither hot nor cold

Sù má naa Wâata - สุมะนาวาต - Central Channel Wind

Tâat Din - ธาตุดิน - Earth element

Tâat bpàt jù bpan - ธาตุปัจจุปัน - Current condition of imbalance

Tâat Fai - ธาตุไฟ - Fire element

Tâat Nám - ธาตน้ำ - Water element

Tâat Lom - ธาตุลม - Wind element

Tâat sà-mùt-tăan - ธาตุสมุฏฐาน -Elemental causative factor

Upekkhā - Equanimity

U-rá Săym-hà - อุระเสมหะ - Mucus of the Chest and Abdomen

Ù-tá-rí-yá - อุทริยะ -New Food

Yòn - หย่อน - Weakened, Depleted, Deficient, slack

Yòo fai - อยู่ไฟ - Time of staying in by the fire during postpartum

Wâata - วาต - Wind. Stems from the Pāli word, vāta.

Wâi Kroo - ไหว้ครู - Ceremony of respect to lineage

Wíp-bpà-rìt - วิปริต - Elemental imbalance

Win-yaana tâat- วิญญาณธาตุ - Consciousness

Wâi Khru

Presenting the Offerings

IMINĀ SAKĀRENA BUDDHAṀ ABHIPŪJAYĀMI,
IMINĀ SAKĀRENA DHAMMAṀ ABHIPŪJAYĀMI,
IMINĀ SAKĀRENA SAṄGHAṀ ABHIPŪJAYĀMI,
(If chanting in a group, ABHIPŪJAYĀMI, is changed to ABHIPUJAYĀMA)

Homage to the Buddha

ARAHAṀ SAMMĀ SAṀBUDDHO BHAGAVĀ,
BUDDHAṀ BHAGAVANTAṀ ABHIVĀDEMI
(bow)

Homage to the Dharma

SVĀKKHĀTO BHAGAVATĀ DHAMMO, DHAMMAṀ NAMASSĀMI
(bow)

Homage to the Sangha

SUPAṬIPANNO BHAGAVATO SĀVAKASAṀGHO,
SAṄGHAṀ NAMĀMI
(bow)

Homage to the Parents

MAYHAṀ MĀTĀ PITŪNAṀ VA,
PĀDE VANDĀMI SĀDARAṀ
(bow)

Homage to Your Teachers

PAÑÑĀVUṬṬHI KARETE TE,
DINNOVĀDE NAMĀMIHAṀ
(bow)

Homage to the Buddha

NAMO TASSA BHAGAVATO ARAHATO SAMMĀ SAṀBUDDHASSA
NAMO TASSA BHAGAVATO ARAHATO SAMMĀ SAṀBUDDHASSA
NAMO TASSA BHAGAVATO ARAHATO SAMMĀ SAṀBUDDHASSA

Taking Refuges

BUDDHAṀ SARAṆAṀ GACCHĀMI
DHAMMAṀ SARAṆAṀ GACCHĀMI
SAṄGHAṀ SARAṆAṀ GACCHĀMI

DUTIYAMPI BUDDHAṀ SARAṆAṀ GACCHĀMI
DUTIYAMPI DHAMMAṀ SARAṆAṀ GACCHĀMI
DUTIYAMPI SAṄGHAṀ SARAṆAṀ GACCHĀMI

TATIYAMPI BUDDHAṀ SARAṆAṀ GACCHĀMI
TATIYAMPI DHAMMAṀ SARAṆAṀ GACCHĀMI
TATIYAMPI SAṄGHAṀ SARAṆAṀ GACCHĀMI

Precepts

PĀṆATIPĀTĀ VERAMAṆĪ SIKKHĀPADAṀ SAMĀDIYĀMI
ADINĀDĀNĀ VERAMAṆĪ SIKKHĀPADAṀ SAMĀDIYĀMIKĀMESU
MICCHĀCĀRĀ VERAMAṆĪ SIKKHĀPADAṀ SAMĀDIYĀMI
MUSĀVĀDĀ VERAMAṆĪ SIKKHĀPADAṀ SAMĀDIYĀMI
SURĀMERAYA MAJJA PAMĀDAṬṬHĀNĀ VERAMAṆĪ SIKKHĀPADAṀ
SAMĀDIYĀMI

Presenting Offerings and
Taking Refuge in the Teachers

YAMAHAṀ GURŪPĀJJHĀYĀCĀRIYAṀ SARAṆAṀ GATO,
IMINĀ SAKKĀRENA GURŪPĀJJHĀYĀCĀRIYAṀ ABHIPŪJAYĀMI

DUTIYAMPI YAMAHAṀ GURŪPĀJJHĀYĀCĀRIYAṀ SARAṆAṀ GATO,
IMINĀ SAKKĀRENA, GURŪPĀJJHĀYĀCĀRIYAṀ ABHIPŪJAYĀMI

TATIYAMPI YAMAHAṀ GURŪPĀJJHĀYĀCĀRIYAṀ SARAṆAṀ GATO,
IMINĀ SAKKĀRENA, GURŪPĀJJHĀYĀCĀRIYAṀ ABHIPŪJAYĀMI

Homage to Jīvaka Kumārabhacca

OṀ NAMO JĪVAKO,
KARUṆIKO SABBA SATTĀNAṀ OSADHA DIBBAMANTAṀ,
PABHĀSO SURIYĀCANDAṀ KUMĀRABHACCO PAKĀSESI
VANDĀMI SIRASĀ AHAṀ
PAṆḌITO SUMEDHASSO AROGĀ SUMANĀ HOMI

Homage to the Reu-sĕe

OṀ NAMASSITVĀ ISĪ SIDDHI,
LOKANĀTHAṀ ANUTTARAṀ,
ISĪ CA BANDHANAṀ SATTHA,
AHAṀ VANDĀMI,
TAṀ ISĪ SIDDHI VESSA

Homages to Personal Deities

Mantra to Invite the Teachers

VANDITVĀ ĀCĀRIYAṀ GURU PĀDAṀ,
ĀGACCHĀYA ĀGACCHĀHI,
SABBA KAMMAṀ PASIDDHI ME,
SABBA ANTARĀYAṀ VINĀSSANTU,
SABBA SIDDHI BHAVANTU ME

Mantra to Receive Blessings from the Teachers

SIDDHI KICCAṀ
SIDDHI KAMMAṀ
SIDDHI KĀRIYA TATHĀGATO
SIDDHI TEJO JAYO NICCAṀ
SIDDHI LĀBHO NIRANTARAṀ
SABBA KAMMAṀ PASIDDHI ME
AHAṀ SIDDHI BHAVANTU ME

Acknowledgment of Faults

KĀYA KAMMAṀ
VACĪ KAMMAṀ
MANO KAMMAṀ
SAÑCICCA DOSAṀ
ASAÑCICCA DOSAṀ
ATĪTA DOSAṀ
ANĀGATA DOSAṀ
PACCUPANNA DOSAṂ
SABBA DOSAṂ
KHAMATHA ME BHANTE

Meditation of Mettā

SABBE SATTĀ
AVERĀ HONTU
ABHYĀPAJJHĀ HONTU
ANĪGHĀ HONTU
SUKHĪ ATTĀNAṂ PARIHARANTU
DUKKHĀ PAMUCCANTU

Meditation of Karunā

SABBE SATTĀ
ALĀBHĀ PAMUCCANTU
AYASĀ PAMUCCANTU
NINDĀ PAMUCCANTU
DUKKHĀ PAMUCCANTU

Meditation of Muditā

SABBE SATTĀ
LADDHASAMPATTITO MĀ VIGACCHANTU
LADDHAYASATO MĀ VIGACCHANTU
LADDHAPASAŃSATO MĀ VIGACCHANTU
LADDHASUKHĀ MĀ VIGACCHANTU

Meditation of Upekkhā

SABBE SATTĀ
KAMMASAKĀ
KAMMA DĀYĀDĀ
KAMMA YONĪ
KAMMA BANDHU
KAMMA PAṬISARAṆĀ
YAṂ KAMMAṂ KARISSANTI
KALYĀṆAṂ VĀ PĀPAKAṂ VĀ
TASSA DĀYĀDĀ BHAVISSANTI

Verses for the Removal of Disease

SAKKATVĀ BUDDHARATANAṂ OSADHAṂ UTTAMAṂ VARAṂHITAṂ
DEVAMANUSSĀNAṂ BUDDHATEJENA SOTTHINĀ NASSANTU PADDAVĀ
SABBE DUKKHĀ VŪPASAMENTU TE

SAKKATVĀ DHAMMARATANAṂ OSADHAṂ UTTAMAṂ
VARAṂPARIḶĀHŪPASAMAṆAṂ DHAMMATEJENA SOTTHINĀNASSANTU
PADDAVĀ SABBE BHAYĀ VŪPASAMENTU TE

SAKKATVĀ SAṄGHARATANAṀ OSADHAṀ UTTAMAṀ VARAṀ
ĀHUNEYYAṀ PĀHUṆEYYAṀ SAṄGHATEJENA SOTTHINĀ
NASSANTU PADDAVĀ SABBE ROGĀ VŪPASAMENTU TE

Verses of Dedication of Merit and Aspiration

IDAṀ ME DĀNAṀ ĀSAVAKKHAYĀVAHAṀ HOTU
IDAṀ ME SĪLAṀ NIBBĀNASSA PACCAYO HOTU
IDAṀ ME BHĀVANAṀ MAGGASSA CA PHALASSA CA PACCAYO HOTU
IDAṀ ME PUÑÑAṀ ĀSAVAKKHAYĀVAHAṀ NIBBĀNAṀ HOTU
IDAṀ ME PUÑÑA BHĀGAṀ SABBA SATTĀNAṀ DEMA

SĀDHU NO BHANTE

Short Wâi Khru

This very short version of the *wâi khru* is for those times when you simply do not have time to do the longer version. It is not meant to replace the longer version in daily life, but to fill in as needed.

NAMO TASSA BHAGAVATO ARAHATO SAMMĀ SAMBHUDDHASSA (3 times)
OṀ NAMO JĪVAKA KUMĀRABHACCA PŪJĀYA *(3 times)*
OṀ NAMO ISĪ MUNI NAMĀMIHAṀ *(3 times)*

General Index

Index of Conditions

Index of Herbs by Common Name

Index of Formulas

FINDHORN PRESS

Life-Changing Books

Consult our catalogue online
(with secure order facility) on
www.findhornpress.com

For information on the Findhorn Foundation:
www.findhorn.org